Jean Piaget: Selected Works

Volume 9

Insights and Illusions
of Philosophy

Jean Piaget

Translated by Wolfe Mays

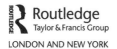
Routledge
Taylor & Francis Group

LONDON AND NEW YORK

First published 1965
by Presses Universitaires de France

English translation first published 1972
by Routledge

Reprinted 1997
by Routledge
2 Park Square, Milton Park, Abingdon, Oxon, OX14 4RN
711 Third Avenue, New York, NY 10017
Routledge is an imprint of the Taylor & Francis Group, an informa business
Transferred to Digital Printing 2006
First issued in paperback 2013
© 1965 Presses Universitaires de France
English translation © 1971 The World Publishing Company

This is a reprint of the 1972 edition

British Library Cataloguing in Publication Data
A catalogue record for this book is available from the British Library

Library of Congress Cataloguing in Publication Data
A catalogue record for this book has been requested

ISBN 13: 978-0-415-16894-6 (Hardback)
ISBN 13: 978-0-415-84513-7 (Paperback)

Publisher's Note
The publisher has gone to great lengths to ensure the
quality of this reprint but points out that some
imperfections in the original may be apparent

Contents

Translator's Introduction   vii

Introduction   xiii

Chapter One

An account of and an analysis of a
    disenchantment   3

Chapter Two

Science and philosophy   39

Chapter Three

The false ideal of a suprascientific
    knowledge   78

*Additional. note on ontology and the
    "inadequacies" of science*   117

Chapter Four

The ambitions of a philosophical
        psychology   122

Chapter Five

Philosophers and problems of fact   165

Conclusion   209

Postscript to the Second Edition   215

Index   233

Translator's Introduction

In THIS valuable book Piaget examines his own philosophical position and compares it with present-day continental philosophical thought. Among other things, he gives the reader a most interesting insight into his own intellectual development and an account of the way in which he finally arrived at his *épistémologie génétique*. Piaget argues that recent continental philosophy has turned away from the empirical world and concentrated on introspective description. He contrasts this with the attitude of most of the great philosophers of the past, who had a decided interest in scientific questions, which affected their mode of thinking. He points out that although philosophy has, among other things, provided a matrix for the development of such sciences as logic, psychology and sociology, it can only give us a "wisdom" and not knowledge in the real sense of the word as we come across it in mathematics and science.

In this connection Piaget examines the attempt of Husserl and others to introduce a mode of knowledge specific to philosophy, and of a higher order logically than that of science. The attempt to look for it in an elementary act of consciousness (i.e. the intentional act), which gives us knowledge of "essences," suffers from the drawback that such acts seem to be a feature of sophisticated adult consciousness. For Piaget, however, adult intellectual activities are conditioned by earlier forms of behavior. He argues that the Achilles heel of philosophers like

Bergson and Husserl, who believe in intuition as an immediate source of knowledge, lies precisely in their neglect of the historical and genetic viewpoints.

Piaget is also concerned with attempts of Maine de Biran, Bergson, Sartre, and Merleau-Ponty to construct a philosophical psychology as opposed to a scientific empirical psychology. He believes that the difference between philosophical psychology and scientific psychology lies neither in the fact that the former concerns itself with "essences" (Husserl), with "irrationality" (Sartre), nor in its use of introspection. He sees the difference as being one rather of method: philosophical psychology neglects objective verification and grounds itself in subjectivity, although claiming to arrive at objective knowledge through intuition.

How far, one may ask, if at all, do Piaget's criticisms of French philosophy and philosophers apply to the Anglo-Saxon philosophical scene? The empirical tradition of British philosophy would, it might be thought, make British philosophers at least sympathetic with Piaget's views, especially as they are somewhat critical of phenomenology and existentialism. Curiously enough, as far as methodology is concerned, the school of conceptual (or linguistic) analysis, which has a substantial following among American philosophers, has certain affinities with that of phenomenology. One finds an acceptance of the view that empirical questions are irrelevant to philosophical ones, and that philosophical discussions of conceptual thinking are concerned with questions of validity and not of origin. Then genetic (historical) dimension is therefore excluded because, as it is sometimes said, it is concerned with the process of discovery and not of justification. The philosopher is interested only in the latter.

One of the points Piaget makes in this book is that philosophers in France represent a social élite, and one which has strongly influenced the pattern of French education. It is interesting to note here that some critics of the Oxford school of linguistic philosophy have pointed out that it, too, is the intellectual expression of an élite. However, its impact on British education is significantly more limited than is the case with philosophy in France. Similarly, Piaget's observations on the university training of French philosophers—that it is divorced from studies of a scientific nature—could equally well apply to the training of many British philosophers. But unlike their French counterparts, they would not be concerned with the arduous study of philosophical texts, but rather with the painstaking study of linguistic usage.

Further, some British philosophers also regard philosophical psychology as a legitimate enterprise distinct from empirical psychology, although they would treat the former in a much more linguistic manner. On this point of view, when the psychologist studies such topics as learning, motivation, perception, etc., he is solely concerned with particular causal or genetic factors. The philosopher's task, on the other hand, is to examine the grammar or logic of the language in which our psychological concepts are expressed. We are told that a subject like physics or psychology has a logical grammar that covers the meaningful use of the terms of the subject, which is not to be determined by empirical investigation. To engage in a philosophical inquiry is then something like doing mathematics or logic.

One may agree that in assessing the correctness of a piece of logical or mathematical reasoning, validity is our sole concern, and that questions of psychological fact—how we actually think —are irrelevant. On the other hand, when we deal with such questions as the nature of learning or concept formation, a reference to psychological facts becomes necessary, as we cannot know what they are by reflection alone. The philosopher's usual counter to this is to say that he is concerned with the logic of learning, thought, etc., and not its psychology. In practice this often comes to discussing the meaning psychological terms have in ordinary discourse, and examining the different ways they are used.

As a result it is assumed that philosophers can talk about the intended meanings, habits, capacities, skills, etc., of human beings without the need to elucidate such questions by reference to psychological research. Such an approach may have had some credence when introspection was the only method used for describing and analyzing psychological phenomena. But have we any grounds today for assuming that our unaided personal observations are incorrigible, as Descartes thought in the case of the _Cogito_, even if they are helped out by an analysis of the language in which they are expressed? It is true that in recent years some philosophers have appealed to behavioral skills rather than introspection in discussing psychological data. However, most of these accounts are highly impressionistic, and are not subject to experimental control or verification. For example, in discussing intellectual skills, there is little or no reference to empirical studies on concept formation.

Piaget's experiments on concept formation have been criticized by some linguistic philosophers on the grounds that they do not show that there is anything wrong with the child's logic, but merely that the child does not know how to use language properly. His lack of understanding of conservation—that objects retain their identity when, for example, their shape is deformed—is due to this and not to a failure to grasp the logical principle of identity. But whether the child can actually understand this concept cannot be decided simply by a reference to normal adult usage. We may have to experiment in order to see in which situations the child can, and in which he cannot, use this concept. For example, when first dealing with a collection of objects the young child cannot distinguish its spatial aspect from its numerical one, so that a change in its shape may lead him to believe that there has been a change in the number of objects. This is not simply a question of failing to understand the use of language. The child still only possesses a rudimentary concept of number, of which invariance is not yet an essential property. Piaget's work shows that our concepts of logic, space, time, number, quantity, etc., are not given readymade as Kant thought, but undergo a process of development.

Philosophers have criticized the empiricists Locke and Mill on the ground that they base their doctrine of concept formation on a muddled notion of abstraction. It is argued that although one could see how concepts like color might be derived from the perceptual facts of abstraction, logical concepts such as negation or disjunction could not be arrived at in this way. They might therefore be tempted to criticize Piaget's views on concept formation on similar grounds. But this would be to overlook that unlike Locke, Piaget does not accept a *tabula rasa* theory of the mind; intellectual operations play an important part in his theory of concept formation—although they are tied to our behavioral activities. Logical concepts like negation or disjunction, as well as mathematical ones like number, are taken as having an operational character, and are not simply discovered as a result of some intellectual intuition.

By and large, then, although Anglo-Saxon linguistic philosophy may seem very different from French philosophical thought, they both seem to have a number of points in common: they believe that philosophical method is radically different from that of empirical science, and also that empirical and genetic questions are irrelevant to philosophical questions. Instead of an appeal to a realm of essences intuitively given, there is a reference to a set of linguistic categories or meanings embedded in our language, which are assumed to be objective in the sense of being nonpsychological. But in both cases we have to explain how we arrive at such norms. This could be done by 1) appealing to intuition or self-evidence, or 2) by verifying that every civilized adult makes use of them. But these are not now simply normative questions to which facts are irrelevant. In 1) we know how people's ideas on self-evidence have changed: Euclid's axioms are a case in point here. In 2) there seems a good deal of evidence to show that such norms are universally applied.

All this should not be taken to mean that Piaget is uninterested in philosophical issues. His thinking, as he points out, has been deeply affected by his earlier philosophical studies, and this has determined the direction taken by his experimental work. Indeed, one cannot fully grasp its scope and purpose unless this fact is appreciated. Philosophy in the past, he tells us, has provided us with "insights," unformalized intuitions, which when made precise and subjected to empirical testing have led to the development of the special sciences. The "illusions" of philosophy, on the other hand, arise from the belief of some philosophers that they are in possession of a special sort of knowledge, given only in reflection.

As we have already noted, Piaget believes that philosophy still has an important part to play in our culture as a "wisdom" —namely, in helping us to coordinate our values, ethical, aesthetic, and social. He makes the interesting point that if Western philosophy had not in its origins been so closely tied up with the development of science, which was not the case with Oriental thought, it would like the latter have followed the path of "wisdom." If, however, we accept such a point of view, one of the prime concerns of philosophy becomes the examination of the important social and moral issues that confront us in the world today. It cannot take up the position that it is neutral as regards these issues.

Wolfe Mays
University of Manchester

Introduction

It WOULD BE pretentious to say that this study is forced upon me as a duty, but perhaps I could say that it is my response to an increasingly pressing need. Its thesis is simple, and in some circles mundane: *viz* that philosophy, as its name implies, is a "wisdom," which man as a rational being finds essential for co-ordinating his different activities, but is not knowledge properly so called, possessing safeguards and methods of verification characteristic of what is usually called "knowledge." But if I have lived comfortably with this belief, as do all those who remain on the fringe of philosophy without being beguiled by it, I now find it necessary to justify this thesis explicitly, in view of the daily errors to which its disregard leads. During my career as a psychologist and epistemologist I have been on excellent terms with philosophers, who have often honored me with their friendship and confidence, which I have greatly appreciated.[1] I have nearly every day been faced with the conflicts that slow down the development of disciplines trying to become scientific. And I have arrived at the conviction that, under the extremely complex set of individual or group factors, university or ideological, epistemological or moral, historical or actual, etc., which enter into each of these conflicts, one always discovers the same problem and under forms that have seemed to me to involve a question

[1] I have even been elected a member of the International Institute of Philosophy, without my having put my name forward as a candidate.

of simple intellectual honesty: under what conditions can one speak of knowledge, and how can one guard against the internal and external dangers that continually threaten it? Whether it is a matter of internal factors or of social constraints, these dangers all occur around the same boundary—one that has been extremely changeable throughout time, but is no less important for the future of knowledge: the boundary that separates verification from speculation.

For someone who constantly comes across this problem in the course of his professional activities, the question whether philosophy has the status of a "wisdom" or of a form of "knowledge" peculiar to itself is no longer an unnecessary or simply a theoretical problem; it is a vital question, since it affects the success or failure of thousands of scholars. Young philosophers, because they are made to specialize immediately on entering the university in a discipline which the greatest thinkers in the history of philosophy have entered only after years of scientific investigations, believe they have immediate access to the highest regions of knowledge, when neither they nor sometimes their teachers have the least experience of what it is to acquire and verify a specific piece of knowledge. This refers then to all who study disciplines concerned directly or indirectly with the mind of man, and whose future career will be constantly conditioned by questions of independence or dependence with respect to philosophy.

One could, of course, be satisfied to deal with this problem in the abstract. Does there or does there not exist a specific mode of knowledge peculiar to philosophy, and which would be distinct from scientific knowledge while possessing norms and a methodology worthy of being called "knowledge"? Assuming an affirmative answer, what are these norms and these criteria, and what are the procedures of verification to which they lead? Are these procedures actually effective and have they ever been successful in putting an end to a dispute by the rejection of a theory, which was then accepted as invalid by all contemporaries, and by adequately justifying this rejection so as to bring about agreement in favor of a successful theory? These will be the kind of problems with which we will certainly have to deal, although we might well have limited ourselves to giving a general and purely epistemological discussion.

But the question is much wider and more serious, as it is sociological and psychological no less than epistemological, and touches the roots of our ideologies just as much and even more than the conditions of our rational activity. In fact, it is not simply "philosophy" with which we are concerned: it is a whole group of extraordinarily powerful and complex historical and social influences, which institutionalize philosophy in both school and university, with all that this involves of tradition, authority, direction of minds, and above all the determination of careers. Further, in many countries philosophy has become a kind of spiritual exercise invested with an aura, which although not exactly sacred gives it a prestige that makes any attempt to question it seem *ipso facto* proof of a narrow positivism or of a congenital lack of understanding.

Nevertheless, philosophy has its *raison d'être*, and one ought to recognize that anyone who has not had some acquaintance with it is hopelessly uneducated. However, this has no bearing on the question of its truth-status. To discuss its scope, and even to question whether it attains knowledge in the full sense of the word, requires "philosophical courage" in the present state of institutions and opinions. For one risks running counter to the most tenacious and deeply rooted forces of the social consciousness as well as each individual consciousness for which philosophical thought has become either a substitute or a necessary support for religion.

If this is so, and if belief in a philosophical "knowledge" is generally connected with a complex set of individual and social motivations, it goes without saying that a writer questioning this feature of knowledge and convinced of the fact that metaphysical thought reduces itself to a wisdom or to a rational faith, is himself necessarily influenced by a multiplicity of motivations. In such a discussion, where everyone is more or less deeply involved, it is impossible to place oneself "above the conflict" and objectivity remains here, to a greater extent than in other spheres, a necessary ideal achieved only with difficulty. It therefore seems to me essential to give the reader the necessary data to enable him to judge my own point of view, and to do this by devoting the first chapter, if not to a confession, at least to a detailed account of a disenchantment that led a former would-be philosopher to become a psychologist and an epistemologist of the development of thought. I am well aware that the self is hateful and that in addition everyone thinks like Gide: ". . . not mine, I would have loved it in another"; but it is only in retracing one's development that one is able to understand the reasons for one's positions, and this can help us to establish their degree of validity.

After this analysis of personal experience, Chapter Two will try to examine the relationships between science and philosophy. We shall try to recall, on the one hand (a commonplace too often forgotten), that the most important philosophical systems of the past have as their starting point their authors' reflections on science or on projects that made new sciences possible. And this accounts, on the other hand, for a general tendency in the history of philosophical ideas: they start off by being neither clearly scientific nor metaphysical, become gradually less metaphysical, and finally give rise to particular autonomous sciences such as logic, psychology, sociology and epistemology, which are increasingly the work of scientists. Reacting against this inevitable differentiation of philosophy into a metaphysics (which is only a "wisdom" or a rational faith but not a mode of knowledge) and the disciplines concerned with knowledge, an entire line of thought originating only in the nineteenth century and having Husserl as its most important contemporary representative, has tended to credit philosophy once again with a specific mode of knowledge that can be labeled suprascientific or parascientific according to one's standpoint. Chapter Three will try to examine the value of such an approach, and in particular the validity of this proposed mode of knowledge. This is "intuition" in its Bergsonian or phenomenological forms, which are, incidentally, contradictory.

We may with advantage study the problem of the possibility of a specifically philosophical and parascientific knowledge in a particular and especially instructive example, *viz* that of so-called philosophical psychology. I do not mean the psychology of the great philosophers of the past, before the establishment of a scientific psychology, but the one that some philosophers wish to found on the fringe of the latter so as to complement and replace it. In Chapter Four we shall examine the question of the validity and the legitimacy of this series of attempts originating with Maine de Biran and ending with those of Sartre and Merleau-Ponty. (Maine de Biran, incidentally, criticized Hume's empiricism and not experimental psychology, which had not yet been founded.)

Finally, in Chapter Five we shall deal with a question that might appear to be secondary, but which remains central for our purpose: whether one is justified in dealing with factual problems by reflection alone.

The aim of this little book is therefore to sound a note of warning and to defend a position. The reader should not look for erudition in its historical allusions nor for depth in the details of the discussion. It does not claim to be more than the testimony of a man who has been tempted by speculation and who almost devoted his life to it, but who has understood its dangers, its illusions, and its many errors and wishes to communicate his experiences and justify his painfully acquired convictions.

Insights and Illusions
of Philosophy

An Account of
and an Analysis of a
Disenchantment

Chapter One

THERE SEEMS little doubt that philosophy has constantly had a twofold aim, that of knowledge and that of the coordination of values; and the different philosophical systems have in different ways sought their more or less complete unification. A first approach is pre-critical: philosophy attains complete knowledge and thus directly coordinates values to particular or scientific knowledge. A second approach characterizes the Kantian critique: specifically philosophical knowledge consists, on the one hand, in determining the limits of all knowledge and, on the other, in giving a theory of scientific knowledge, and the establishment of such limits leaves the field free for the coordination of values. While not claiming that this account is exhaustive, we list a third group of solutions; this exhibits two tendencies. On the one hand, certain branches of philosophy are separated, i.e. those which have become autonomous disciplines, such as psychology, sociology, logic, and increasingly epistemology, which is becoming part of science. On the other hand, values are coordinated by reflection. This latter proceeds (in a countless variety of ways) by a critical examination of science and by looking for a specific mode of knowledge; and this is either immanent in this critique, or is boldly established on the fringe of scientific knowledge, or above it.

(A) When an adolescent approaches philosophy, he is in general largely motivated by the need for the coordination of values: to reconcile faith and science or reason, etc. His scientific knowledge is restricted to certain summary results learned at school, but he has as yet no idea about research as such nor about the complex conditions necessary for the establishment of truth, for these are realities which only personal and lived experience enables us to understand. Since all teaching, with very few exceptions, is based on verbal transmission and reflection, the adolescent readily accepts a mode of philosophical knowledge based on his reflection alone, and he cannot but be thrilled thus to discover simultaneously an approach to the higher truths, much more central than the simpler truths given by everyday teaching, and an answer to the vital questions he asks with regard to the highest values in which he believes. Either he decides to devote himself to philosophy, or he will keep its permanent imprint and may set himself new problems if he later studies borderline subjects.

I decided to devote myself to philosophy as soon as I was introduced to the subject. But by an accident that influenced my subsequent development considerably, I already had at this time specific interests persistent enough to become permanent. Like many children I was fascinated by natural history, and at the age of eleven I had the good fortune to become the *famulus*, as he called me, of an old zoologist, Paul Godot, who directed the Museum at Neuchâtel solely on his own resources. In exchange for my small services, he introduced me to malacology and gave me a number of shells of land and freshwater mollusks with which I made my own collection at home. When he died in 1911, I published at the age of fifteen several notes by way of a supplement to his *Catalogue of Neuchâtel Mollusks* as well as on alpine mollusks, which much interested me in their variability of adaptation to altitude.

It is in this context that I discovered philosophy. My father, who was an historian but did not believe in historical knowledge, was delighted that I did not follow in his footsteps (an excellent example of self-sacrifice). But my godfather, a man of letters without children who took an interest in me, was alarmed by this exclusive specialization and one summer invited me to stay at his house on the shores of Lake Annecy, his intention being to have me read and to explain to me Bergson's *Évolution créatrice*. This was a tremendous experience, and for two equally strong reasons, both of which merged with those basic interests that impel adolescents toward philosophy.

The first of these reasons was cognitive: it was to find the answer to the great problems met with during my intellectual development. Deeply interested in biology as I was, but understanding nothing of mathematics, physics, nor of the logical reasoning they presuppose, I was fascinated by the dualism of the *élan vital* and of matter falling back on itself, or by that of the intuition of duration and of intelligence unable to understand life because its logical and mathematical structures are oriented in the direction of inert matter. I discovered a philosophy answering exactly to my then intellectual interests.

On the other hand, I was brought up in the Protestant faith by a believing mother, whereas my father was a nonbeliever, and I was therefore already acutely aware of the conflict of science and religion. The reading of Auguste Sabatier's *L'évolution des dogmes*, which I found in my father's library, had convinced me of the symbolic character of expressions of faith, but I still believed without finding a satisfying formula in historical relativity. Reading Bergson was again a revelation from this second point of view: in a moment of enthusiasm close to ecstatic joy, I was struck by the certainty that God is Life, under the form of the *élan vital*, and my biological interests provided me at the same time with a small sector of study. Internal unity was thus achieved in the direction of an immanentism which has long satisfied me. To say that over the years it has taken other, increasingly rational forms would be to anticipate.

On returning to school my decision was made: I would devote my life to philosophy, whose central aim I saw as the reconciliation between science on the one hand, and religious values on the other. But I came in contact with a teacher who strongly influenced me, although in two opposing directions. On the one hand, he got me to appreciate rational values, and on the other, he influenced me indirectly by gradually making me doubt the value of the profession of philosophy. This was the logician Arnold Reymond, who began his career at Neuchâtel. His inaugural lecture, at which I was present before being his pupil at the gymnasium (lycée), was a critique of the work of Bergson, which at first made me want to object to his essentially mathematical approach.

I had been struck by a remark of Bergson that appeared to give me a guiding thread for the start of my philosophico-biological studies. This was his surprise at the disappearance of the problem of "kinds" in modern philosophy in favor of the problem of laws. The curriculum of the Neuchâtel gymnasium was then so liberal, under the guidance of an exceptionally intelligent director, that one found time to work, if one may put it thus. While continuing my articles on malacology (among others on Lake Annecy!), I began to write "my" philosophy. After having read James, I produced an *Outline of Neo-Pragmatism*, which took account of the rationalist criticism of Reymond but remained under Bergson's influence, and in which I tried to show that there exists a logic of action distinct from mathematical logic. Then, turning to the problem of "kinds," I wrote a tome (happily without contemplating speedy publication) on *Realism and Nominalism in the Life-Sciences*, in which I put forward a kind of holism, or philosophy of wholes: the reality of species, genera, etc., and, of course, of the individual as an organized system. My original intention was to create a science of kinds—neither more nor less—which would be distinct from science as a lawlike endeavor, and would thus justify the Bergsonian dualism between the vital and mathematics, a dualism in which I still believed. But with the first written accounts of this, which I made for Reymond (who followed my youthful enterprise with patience and admirable kindness), I was naïvely surprised to discover that my problem was not far removed from that of classes in logic, and that my logic of life could easily fit into that of the great Aristotle, whose concept of form was precisely conceived as governing thought while at the same time corresponding to the structures of the organism! This meant the end of my belief in the Bergsonian opposition of the vital to the logico-mathematical and I was ready to follow Reymond's instruction in logic and mathematical philosophy. I even began to understand mathematics through the latter, and by reading La Vallée-Poussin's set-theory. Subsequently, I carried out some biometrical researches on the variability of my alpine mollusks, and this finally convinced me.

(B) Arnold Reymond was a philosopher by inclination, and he remained for me the fullest and most admirable example of a thinker. He approached no question, intellectual, practical, economic or any other, without making it yield considerations so surprisingly general as to lead on to the great metaphysical questions. A former theologian who had given up the pastorate for reasons of conscience, his interests remained centered on the problems of the relations between science and faith, but his considerable studies in the field of mathematical philosophy made him also an authority on epistemological matters. Finally, his studies on Greek science bore witness to a profound and judicious use of the historico-critical method. It was therefore with the greatest confidence that I let him guide me into following an essentially philosophical career, and to specializing in biological philosophy. When I entered the university, it was hence understood that I would take my *license* and my doctorate in biology, while following Reymond's course in the Faculty of Letters, and that I would then work on a thesis with him after complementary examinations in philosophy.

Finding philosophy everywhere, Reymond had no qualms in taking on the crushing syllabus for which he was then responsible: history of philosophy, general philosophy, philosophy of science, psychology, and sociology. (At Neuchâtel there were not at that time separate chairs for the last two disciplines.) With his help I made such progress in epistemology that after a study on the epistemology of biology as a science, I began to contemplate, in keeping with my former interests, a more long-winded work on the theory of knowledge in general, but looked at from a biological standpoint: in other words, a study similar to that of Spencer, but without its empiricist perspective and in line with our present knowledge in epistemology and biology. But for this I required some understanding of psychology, and it is here that slight differences of opinion began to show themselves between Reymond and myself.

I had arrived at two ideas central for my point of view and which, moreover, I have never given up. The first is that since every organism has a permanent structure, which can be modified under the influence of the environment but is never destroyed as a structured whole, all knowledge is always *assimilation* of a datum external to the subject's structure. This view is opposed to Le Dantec's, who, though making biological assimilation in its widest sense the keystone of his doctrine, regarded knowledge as an organic "imitation" of objects. The second is that the normative factors of thought correspond biologically to a necessity of *equilibrium* by self-regulation: thus logic would in the subject correspond to a process of equilibrium.

But I, a zoologist working in the field or in the laboratory, began (very slowly, alas) to feel that an idea is only an idea and a fact is simply a fact. To see my teacher treat all ideas as if they were never more than a question of metaphysics made me uneasy. I began to feel that in order to analyze the relations between knowledge and organic life it would perhaps be useful to study a little experimental psychology, to which Reymond replied that excellent minds like those of his friends Claparède or Languier de Bancels had allowed themselves to be beguiled by it, but at the price of increasingly wasted time or increasingly limited problems, whereas a well-directed reflection . . . I did, however, observe that this well-directed reflection could lead to indiscretions. Reymond had, for example, been very opposed to the theory of relativity, which ran counter to his need for the absolute, particularly in the domain of time. He had therefore over a long period reflected on the problem and planned a formal refutation of Einstein's view that time was relative to velocity, although his pupils and friends tried to restrain his zeal (especially G. Juvet, who after a period of skepticism became a convinced relativist). When Bergson later published *Durée et simultanéité*, Reymond was distressed at not having anticipated him . . . then most relieved at having been won over by counsels of prudence when he saw how this little book was received by specialists in the field. Another simple example: he had given and published a lecture on *The Instinct of Imitation*, a delightful lecture, but one in which he had forgotten to inform himself about the learning process characterizing this function, which has nothing instinctive about it. A trifle certainly, but where is the boundary between that on which reflection may pronounce with certainty, and that which the facts compel us to amend?

A break in my studies and some months spent in the mountains had forced me to make up my mind. There was as yet no question of my choosing between philosophy and psychology, but only of deciding whether it was necessary for a serious study of epistemology to spend several semesters studying psychology. These months of leisure naturally revived my desire to write: I prepared a paper on the equilibrium between the whole and the parts in an organized structure (although as yet completely unaware of *Gestalt* theory), and on the correspondence between normative obligation and equilibrium. But as I had doubts, I did not wish to present this as a "serious" text, and I incorporated it in a kind of philosophical novel (and Reymond then published a severe criticism of it!).

After my doctorate I spent several months at Zurich studying psychology with G. E. Lipps and Wreschner and some psychiatry with Bleuler, but without making much headway. Then I left for Paris, determined to combine researches in psychology with the teaching of Brunschvicg and Lalande. I had the extraordinary luck to work almost alone in Binet's laboratory, in a school where I was given a free hand, and to be entrusted with a study aiming in principle to restandardize intelligence tests, but which in fact allowed me to analyze the different levels of the logic of classes and relations in child thought. Lalande was willing to read and approve these results before publication, and I finally had the feeling of having found a way of reconciling epistemological research with respect for the facts, and a field of studies intermediary between the domain of psychological development and the problems of normative structures.

But because of this I did not feel myself any the less a philosopher, and when Claparède offered me a post at the *Institut J. J. Rousseau*, I happily developed my researches there, having had for long the impression of working at subjects on the fringe of psychology. My first studies on the logic of the child were given a friendly reception by Brunschvicg and Lalande. Reymond regarded them as a kind of extension or parallel of the historico-critical method applied, as Brunschvicg said, to the "ages of intelligence" instead of to history. I was just as pleased, but a little more surprised, by the friendly response of psychologists (P. Janet, *et al.*). However, when Reymond left Neuchâtel for Lausanne, I did not hesitate to take his advice and put my name forward to succeed him in 1925, although I had still not undertaken the projected doctorate under him. I was nevertheless appointed in view of my work,[1] my only regret being that it was no longer possible to submit a thesis in philosophy, since I held the chair.

I say all this in order to show that I did not begin my career with an unfavorable prejudice toward philosophy. True, in 1929 I rejoined a Faculty of Science and taught, in Geneva, at first the history of scientific thought then experimental psychology; but I did this without dogmatic prejudice and simply in order to find a more extensive field of experience.

(C) All the same, the result was a kind of progressive disenchantment, and it is important to analyze the reasons for it. There were at least three. The first is that nothing is more pro-

---

[1] I had been appointed to the chair of philosophy with a combined teaching load of twelve hours! However, I immediately asked a colleague appointed to teach aesthetics for two hours, to take over the teaching of the history of philosophy, which certainly attracted me, but the serious teaching of which might have prevented me from continuing with my studies.

vocative of self-examination than the start of a teaching career in philosophy, where one is completely free to develop no matter what idea, but where one succeeds much better than one's audience in achieving a clear awareness of degrees of certainty. No great lucidity is required to discover with what ease one can contrive the presentation or justification of a thesis, so that from being at first doubtful it seems to become self-evident. Nor is it difficult to see that self-reflection presents exactly the same dangers. P. Janet had clearly shown that internal reflection is socially internalized conduct: a discussion or deliberation with oneself, such as one has learned to conduct with others, and in the course of which the same skills can well be employed to persuade oneself as are used in persuading others. The situation is in reality worse, for in putting an argument across to an opponent in a discussion (or in a theoretical exposition before an audience) one is very conscious of one's own strategies, whereas, when one convinces oneself by reflection, there is the constant risk of being the victim of one's unconscious desires. In the case of philosophical reflection these unconscious desires are connected with one's deepest intellectual and moral values, which are or appear to be the most disinterested, so that the more altruistic the cause the greater the risk of self-persuasion, to the evident detriment of objectivity and of the truth-value of the results obtained.

The first reason for my growing disaffection with the traditional methods of philosophy was caused in the main by the conflict, which I felt within myself, between the habits of verification of the biologist and the psychologist, and speculative reflection, which constantly tempted me, but which could not possibly be submitted to verification, as I could see increasingly clearly. Although speculative reflection is a fertile and even necessary heuristic introduction to all inquiry, it can only lead to the elaboration of hypotheses, as sweeping as you like, to be sure, but as long as one does not seek for verification by a group of facts established experimentally or by a deduction conforming to an exact algorithm (as in logic), the criterion of truth can only remain subjective, in the manner of an intuitive satisfaction, of "self-evidence," etc. When it is a question of metaphysical problems involving the coordination of values judged to be of essential importance, problems which thus introduce factors of conviction or faith, speculative reflection remains the only method possible; but remaining bound up with the whole personality of the thinker, it can only lead to a wisdom or rational faith, and is not knowledge from the point of view of objective or interindividual criteria of truth. When it is a question, on the other hand, of the more delimited or delimitable problems of epistemology, then an appeal to facts or to logico-mathematical deduction becomes possible: the historico-critical method of my teachers Brunschvicg and Reymond, the psychogenetic analyses of the formation of concepts and operations, the logical analysis of the foundations of mathematics, provide methods of testing that individual reflection is unable to provide.

In short, two ever deepening convictions were forced on me at the beginning of my teaching career. One is that there is a kind of intellectual dishonesty in making assertions in a domain concerned with facts, without a publicly verifiable method of testing, and in formal domains without a logistic one. The other is that the sharpest possible distinction should at all times be made between personal improvisation, the dogma of a school or whatever is centered on the self or on a restricted group, and, on the other hand, the domains in which mutual agreement is possible, independently of metaphysical beliefs or of ideologies. Whence the essential rule of only asking questions in such terms that verification and agreement is possible, a truth only existing as a truth from the moment in which it has been verified (and not simply accepted) by other investigators.

My second reason for disaffection may well appear odd to pure philosophers. It refers to something which from the psychosociological point of view is very significant: this is the surprising dependence of philosophical ideas in relation to social or even political change. At that time I knew nothing of Marxism, nor of its thesis about the relations between idealism and bourgeois ideology; the very important works of Lukacs and Goldmann on the relations between philosophy and class-consciousness had not yet appeared. I shall therefore not be referring here to this aspect of things. But I was very much struck, after the First World War (and still more so after the Second) by the repercussions that the social and political instability then prevailing in Europe had on the intellectual climate, and this naturally led me to doubt the objective and universal value of the philosophical standpoints adopted in such conditions.

In my peaceful little country, which is relatively isolated from political and social upheavals, numerous signs indicated this dependence of ideas on social factors. For example, Protestant thought, which had been surprisingly liberal before and immediately after the war, began to show signs of a narrow and aggressive Calvinism, which was of great interest for the sociologist but most of all for philosophers (who began, however, to be affected by it particularly later on). Before the war, a highly intelligent theologian, Emile Lombard, had defended a distinguished thesis on *La glossolalie chez les premiers chrétiens,* which was a fine psychological study, suggested by the researches of Flournoy (in "a case of somnambulism with glossolalia") and contained an excellent analysis of pathological phenomena which had characterized revivalism in Wales. In 1925 the same writer was fiercely Calvinist and thought only of defending Western civilization against the dangers of "bolshevism" both externally and . . . internally (and thus including liberal Protestantism!). At the end of the war, the Protestant students had asked me to give two or three lectures on immanentism and religious faith. These were in a Brunschvicgian style (except that, being a biologist, I have always believed in the "external world") and were very sympathetically received: a few years later I would have been booed.

In the specifically philosophical field, I had many discussions between 1925 and 1929 with my colleague Pierre Godot, who taught the history of philosophy with much subtlety and with whom I got on very well, despite his right-wing political opinions. He used to confide in me that by personal temperament he was tempted by a certain historical relativism, and that in particular my psychogenetic point of view in epistemology would suit him very well if he were to let himself be guided solely by intellectual considerations, but that socially these views are dangerous because man has need of stable and absolute realities. He often quoted E. Lombard as a model of a return to wisdom after an excess of religious psychology. I am sure that if he had published more, this kind of confession would certainly have been disguised under all sorts of seemingly objective justifications. My friend Gustave Juvet, mathematician, astronomer, and occasional philosopher, justified his Platonism in the name of mathematics,[2] but I knew well enough that it was a kind of affective halo. He was "anti-genetic because there must be a permanent order in intelligence as in society."

While in French-speaking Switzerland a Maurassian stream of ideas was thus unsettling the metaphysics of élite individuals, who had, however, been brought up as democratic Protestants. German-speaking Switzerland was the scene of intellectual events no less instructive for me and even emotionally disturbing as far as the relations between philosophy and psychology are concerned. One of the signs of the social malaise in Germany at this time and which came to a head with Hitler, was a kind of romanticism of the Geist, resulting, among many other things, in a strong opposition between Geisteswissenschaften and Naturwissenschaften. This led to a disapproval of experimental psychology, although it had largely originated in that country. (It was subsequently almost eliminated from German universities under the Hitler regime and suffered the same fate in Italy under Mussolini. It is now once more flourishing in these two countries.) The intellectuals of German-speaking Switzerland were very courageously anti-Nazi during the Second World War, but during the decades that preceded it they failed to perceive the relations between this new Germanic tendency

[2] See his fine book on La structure des nouvelles théories physiques, Alcan (1933).

to proscribe scientific research in the domain of mind and the temporary pathological situation of German social life and thought; and so they followed the movement. At the University of Zurich, where the psychology chairs had had eminent occupants, Lipps and Wreschner were not replaced and instead appointments were made in the philosophy of mind.[3] The situation at the University of Berne has now been remedied with the excellent teaching of R. Meili, but for a long time a native of Italian-speaking Switzerland taught a kind of Italian neo-Hegelianism under the name of psychology. Inspired by Gentile and adapted to his style, it was, if I may venture to speak as a psychologist, a model of "autistic" philosophy. At Bâle, P. Häberlin, who had started his career with some intelligent studies in child-psychology, later took up a philosophical anthropology that aimed explicitly at replacing psychology. The Lucerne Foundation, which Häberlin directed, awarded me a prize at the beginning of my researches, but toward the 1930's it refused to distribute one of my books to its members, because "the works of Piaget explicitly contradict those of Häberlin," as P. Bovet, who had asked for a copy, was told.

I apologize for speaking only of Switzerland, but these are facts that greatly impressed me at the time and which, moreover, are all the more instructive, since they concern a small country both independent of and yet contributing to three great cultures. Such facts (and many others observed in countries of which I have less right to speak) have convinced me of the close relation that exists betwteen philosophical thought and the underlying social factors; and perhaps the fact that at the time I

---

[3] At Zurich, psychology is severely limited to either the psychoanalytical or philosophical domains: on one occasion B. Inhelder, looking over the "Psychology" shelf in a large university library asked, "You have nothing on intelligence?" and received the following answer: "Oh! you put intelligence under psychology? We never knew where exactly to classify it and have placed it under medicine!" All praise, therefore, to the psychiatrists; and take heed those of you who never consult them on the imprudent pretext that the possession of a clear intelligence does not give rise to any nosological questions—as though this were not a disturbing symptom from the Jungian point of view. . . .

c

was teaching, among other subjects, sociology, helped to strengthen this conviction in me. Speculative reflection does not therefore run the risk of neglecting verification simply as a result of subjective improvisation. The human person only succeeds in being productive in symbiosis with others, even in the solitude of mental work. Thus it follows that either we must adopt systematically a method of cooperation as in science, where truth is only achieved as a result of verifications carried out by many co-workers in the field of facts and that of deduction; or else the self, believing itself free, is unconsciously affected by the suggestions or the pressures of the social group—this we cannot accept, for sociocentrism, like egocentrism, is diametrically opposed to rational cooperation.

(D) The third reason for my disenchantment with regard to philosophy is at the same time the main reason for my becoming a professional psychologist, albeit one with interests centered on problems of epistemology, rather than a philosopher temporarily occupied with psychological verifications before going on to outline a genetic epistemology. The third reason has been the reaction of a certain number of philosophers, whose interpretations or criticisms gave me the impression that we no longer speak the same language; not indeed because theirs was critical (we have just seen that criticism is an essential function of rational cooperation), but because it seemed to me to indicate an attempt having little validity on the part of philosophical judgment to meddle in the field of scientific research. I will give only two illustrations, the second of which is crucial.

When the philosopher I. Benrabi made a survey of philosophical tendencies among French-speaking philosophers, he gave me the honor of mentioning me, although not of discussing my work, and classified me as a positivist. Before the survey was published, I mentioned to him that I did not consider myself a positivist, except insofar as I dealt with facts "positive" if you like, but which appear to me to refute positivism. "Positivism," I said to him, "is a certain form of epistemology which neglects or underestimates the activity of the subject in **favor** of verification or the generalization of the verified laws. However, all my studies have demonstrated to me the role of the subject's activities and the rational necessity of causal explanation. I feel myself much closer to Kant or Brunschvicg than to Comte, and close to Meyerson, whose arguments against positivism I constantly verify (putting aside the identification). "Yes, but you do not believe in philosophy." "Not yours, but there are many others, and I believe as much as you in the major importance of epistemological problems." "But you deal with them in the field of scientific inquiry." "Certainly, but positivism is specifically a doctrine intended to limit science, to assign definite boundaries to it, while for nonpositivist scientists, science is indefinitely open and can inquire into any problem, provided a method can be found about which scientists agree." But it all made no difference: I remained a positivist and proved myself true to type by challenging my opponent's belief in his ability to discover the truth by simply meditating in his study by the light of his own reason. And unhappily, this kind of dialogue of the deaf has continued all my life. Sometimes, however, more amusingly, as at Barcelona where I read on the visiting-card which a professor had presented to me: "Senor X. Cathedratico de psychologia superior." "Why higher?" I asked frankly. "Because it is not experimental. . . ." His colleagues' smiles were well worth seeing.

Prescribing norms to a scientific investigator is an even more serious interference in his affairs than any crude attempt at classifying him. This, of course, is a natural tendency of philosophers, since the essential function of philosophy is precisely the coordination of values. In fact, I was becoming more and more convinced that this is its sole valid function. And when someone who is a metaphysician by inclination manages to reconcile the norms of his knowledge with those of his faith, whatever it may be, it is natural that he should wish to start a school or at least to propagate his convictions. The point where this action begins to become questionable morally (solely from the point of view of intellectual honesty, of course) and not only from a rational standpoint is, it seems to me, that at which scientific inquiry begins. There is no sharp division between scientific and philosophical problems, but scientific problems are more strictly delimited, the purpose of this delimitation being to state them in such a way as to allow experimental and algorithmic testing. Both these modes of testing, as well as this delimitation, presuppose a preliminary training, *i.e.* a technical skill that is acquired only with difficulty; and above all they presuppose clear-cut norms common to the body of scientific investigators (of all philosophical opinions), and formulated as a very function of the inquiry. When an individual metaphysician (and there are still some, since there exists an indefinite multiplicity of schools and positions), having no other training than a perfect knowledge of philosophical authors and that afforded by his personal meditation, however extensive, undertakes to prescribe norms to a scientific discipline, one cannot but fear some abuse of privilege. This is precisely the experience I began to have and which I have had repeatedly since, and nothing has made me more conscious of my community of interests with the worldwide movement of scientific psychology.

I often met philosophers of all levels who wished to subordinate my norms to those of "the" philosophy. They would adduce two arguments, which were, however, reducible to each other. The first, which was used in the main by young philosophers, was to argue as follows: psychology is a particular science and is subject to the laws of knowledge; philosophy is the science of the foundations of all the sciences, and of the general laws of knowledge; there is therefore a vicious circle in trying to understand anything about knowledge by means of psychological studies, since as a psychologist you are subject to the norms of philosophy. Incidentally, this was before Husserl's phenomenology became known and therefore in no way refers to the Husserlian claim to limit the domain of psychology to the spatio-temporal "world," a question to which we will return (Chapter Three). It was therefore easy to reply that "the" philosophy has merely an ideal existence and that as the norms of any system whatever, such as empiricism, can be shown to contradict those of some other system, such as Kantianism, it was certainly permissible: 1) to try to discover the norms with which subjects of every age comply spontaneously (information in no way yielded by "philosophical reflection," centered as it is on the self or on the social group, and which, on the contrary, presupposes an objective psychological analysis); and 2) to comply as a psychologist only with the norms of psychological inquiry, which the philosopher ought to take account of instead of prescribing them, for one only constructs the "Poetic Arts" after poetry.

The second argument, which H. Mieville has developed since then in Dialectica [4] (against Gouseth and myself), was more profound. "You claim to find evidence for an evolution of norms," I was told, "even for a 'directed' evolution, or one that is oriented toward certain structures in the form of a progressive equilibrium. But this inquiry is carried out by means of certain norms common to all minds (including yours), such as the principle of identity. There is thus an absolute, which is a condition of all relativism even if it is systematic; and it is this absolute with which philosophy concerns itself and on which you are thus dependent, whether you like it or not." I answered that I have nothing against the absolute except a kind of individual or idiosyncratic distrust, which I have a professional duty not to accept at its face value; and that if this absolute exists, I will certainly find it in the facts. But I asked above all (as I had asked myself constantly during the period when I still believed in philosophy) by means of what method and in the name of what norms of truth one discovers reflectively the common and absolute Norms of Truth; but here again there is a vicious circle and one just as flagrant when proceeding by objective and not reflective analysis. There are only three possible methods.

1) There is first of all intuition, or self-evidence, but one knows what this yardstick is worth, since all history (and phi-

---

[4] See Dialectica, 1953 and 1954.

losophy as well as science) show their variations: intuitive self-
evidence simply means subjective certainty; [5]

2) To escape from this there is then the verification that
every normal being, adult and civilized, thinks according to such
a norm (where one does not refer to "every human being");

3) There is finally the necessary deduction: every thinking
being ought to apply such a norm if he wants to arrive at truth
(and Lalande added, he ought to do all this if he thinks honestly).

Now, how does the philosopher apply methods 2 and 3? As
far as method 2 is concerned, which raises a question of *fact*
as against method 3, I was increasingly struck, and in some
cases amazed, by the remarkable contrast between the statements of principle made by honest and convinced men, for
whom the cult of norms seemed to form the chief spiritual exercise, and the ease with which they decided formidable questions of fact ("every man thinks that . . ."), as if the verification
of a fact and above all the assertion of its generality did not presuppose the same normative honesty as a judgment concerned
with ideas. Thinking this over, I saw that this was the deplor-
able result of the completely formal education received by philosophy students, based on a respect for texts and a complete
neglect of the way in which facts are established. On the other
hand, any laboratory worker knows that after having worked for
months on the description of quite a small phenomenon, he
finds himself faced, after the publication of his results, with the
possibility that fresh studies made by other investigators will
either verify his results or, on the contrary, demonstrate something else. But without having gone through this experience,
the philosopher who cheerfully proclaims the universality of
the principle of identity, could still ask what this assertion means
factually: whether it concerns a moral law that we respect but
without it ever being completely applied, a syntactic law charac-

[5] We will come back to transcendental intuition (Chapter Three),
which does not possess any method other than reflection even when it is
termed eidetic.

teristic of the speech of man, a law of behavior concerning the whole individual, a cognitive law covering perception as well as intelligence, or a law specific to intelligence, but starting from which level? At that time I observed children who when shown a row of counters said: "There are 7 of them." "And like this (spacing them out a little)?" "A few more." "They have not been added to?" "No." "Then are there only 7 (without counting)?" "No, 8 or 9." "But where do they come from?" "You have made it longer." When the same child one or two years later says: "You have only made it longer, but there are still 7," one can certainly speak of identity, but when 7 counters become 8 or 9, like a piece of elastic 7 cm. in length that stretches to 8 or 9 cm., is it the same principle of identity or a somewhat different principle? My philosopher friends were ready with their answers. I have, however, forgotten which.[6]

In short, method 2 presupposes psychology not as a doctrine, but as the only objective method of investigation as soon as one refers to subjects other than oneself.

As for method 3 it presupposes, of course, logic. But we all know that as a result of the work of mathematicians and logicians, logic has become an independent discipline, presupposing refined techniques greatly neglected in my own country until recently. We are therefore once again far from the reflective analysis proceeding by simple meditation. But as logic has become diversified into a number of logics, consistent, moreover, with one another, each is alone too poor for reason to be based

[6] I remember, on the contrary, a lively discussion I had at Cambridge, around 1926–27 (after a lecture on a similar topic) with the distinguished philosopher G. E. Moore, who then edited *Mind*: the question is of no interest at all, he said, in substance, because the philosopher is concerned with true ideas, while the psychologist feels a sort of vicious and incomprehensible attraction for the study of false ideas! To this I replied that the history of science is full of ideas which we judge today to be false: "How do you know, therefore, that your true ideas will not at a later date be judged to be inadequate? This would seem to point to the existence of progressive approximations, therefore of a development." "That's all the same to me, since my specific work is only concerned with the search for the true."

on it and together they are too complex to give a unique answer: the problem is therefore once again far from being solved.

(E) In 1929 I returned to Geneva and was attached to the Faculty of Science (which has included experimental psychology since 1890, the date of the foundation of the chair and the laboratory by Theodore Flournoy). I felt freed from philosophy and more determined than ever to study epistemological structures using the historico-critical approach, the logistic if possible, and above all the psychogenetic one. I began the study of operational structures, properly so called, in mental development (with A. Szeminska, and then with B. Inhelder), and I produced a kind of logical formalization applicable to the collected facts (*Classes, relations et nombres*, Vrin, 1942). These different studies having interested psychologists, I no longer felt myself to be as I had previously, a kind of free-lance, suspect but tolerated,[7] and when I succeeded Claparède, who died in 1940, I used the equipment of his laboratory in order to conduct a series of researches on perceptual development, which completed my work on the psychology of the child.

Nonetheless, my relationships with my philosophical colleagues of the Faculty of Letters were excellent. H. Reverdin had written a thesis on James, was an admirer of Höffding, and sympathized with my interests (it was he, when I started at Geneva, who had urged me to write a book on *The Moral Judgment of the Child*). C. Werner bore no ill will to experimental psychology, while believing in a philosophical psychology as a necessary complement, but he based the latter on problems of freedom and the immortal soul with a superb detachment with regard to questions of fact and epistemology.

After the 1939–45 war, philosophical psychology, whose value had always appeared to me comparable with that of German nineteenth-century *Naturphilosophie*, revived under a new form due to phenomenology and existentialism. I will not speak here of Husserl, of whom I have only seen later in reading him

---

[7] It must be remembered that I have never in my life passed an examination in psychology, except at the *bachot*, together with philosophy.

that he was worthy of the greatest respect, even if we translate his logicism inspired by Frege into a completely different language. What struck me at the start in considering the phenomenological psychology of his followers, for which he is certainly not responsible, is the similarity of these postwar movements with those after the 1914–18 war: the need for a philosophical anthropology, due to varied social reasons, but comparable mutatis mutandis to that which Bergsonism had satisfied twenty-five or thirty years earlier. To see Sartre's joy in finally attaining reality by breaking away from "Brunschvicgian idealism," without seeming to realize that this "idealism" was really an anti-a-priorist and anti-empiricist theory of science, makes one feel that this attainment of reality and existence is directed toward completely other ends than the genuine cognitive (God be praised, moreover, for Sartre is an admirable playwright). As for Merleau-Ponty's Phénoménologie de la Perception, this essay of pure reflection, which only bases itself with regard to facts on already known studies (Gestalt Psychology), has made a bewildering impression on me, which was increased when I read later in the Bulletin de psychologie of the way in which he understood and discussed my studies in perception in his lectures at the Sorbonne.[8] I find it difficult to understand how a writer who so admirably analyzes the "ambiguities" of consciousness and subjectivity has not as a result of this analysis got out of subjectivity, if only by discovering how the primitive and lived experiences studied by him are always the product of a history that includes subjectivity and does not result from it.

Some years later, when Merleau-Ponty was appointed to the Collège de France, I was called to succeed him in the chair he occupied in the Faculty of Letters at the Sorbonne. This was, apart from the joy which this great honor gave me, one of the greatest surprises of my life. I do not refer to the delightful wel-

[8] A single example, in connection with seriation: Merleau-Ponty criticizes me for considering it "as a sum" when it forms "a new whole," Bul. de Psychol., 1965, p. 185. This is a point I constantly make, since the concept of operational wholes superimposing themselves on perceptual wholes is basic to my interpretations. . . .

come of the students, some of whom asked if this Swiss would
know French (nor do I refer to my first correction of the examination answers, for some candidates, not noticing that the professor had changed, explained that Piaget had understood nothing whatever, "as M. Merleau-Ponty has demonstrated": I,
nevertheless, raised their marks). I refer to the reasons for this
appointment, for I have never known whether they rested on
a misunderstanding: I have, in fact, been welcomed in the most
friendly manner, and the most moving for me, by my new colleagues of the philosophy section, but as if I bore the stamp of
the psychologist-philosopher! I kept up my teaching in the
Faculty of Science at Geneva, and I had at last published my
Introduction à l'épistémologie génétique, in which I presented
this method of inquiry as independent of all philosophy. But
G. Bachelard did not appear to bear me any ill will, and my
other colleagues had undoubtedly not read this much-too-large
three-volume work.

But I have not for that matter become a philosopher again,
and I have, on the contrary, acquired during my years at the
Sorbonne, an entirely new experience of the dangers of philosophy for psychological and sociological research. I can speak of
it now without excessive caution, for I have found these dangers
within one of the finest teaching centers in Europe, due not to
the men, who were admirable, but to the institutions. I therefore discovered in France a sociological verification, so to speak,
of my hypotheses, and no longer by means of individual observations.

French psychology has an honored past and occupies at the
moment a very important position. Its pre-eminence is in particular to be seen in the International Union of Scientific Psychology, to which all the psychological societies in the world
belong, and whose first president was H. Pieron. However, if
we compare the official and university position of psychological
studies in France and in countries like Great Britain, Germany,
Italy, Belgium, etc. (without referring to the U.S.A. or USSR),
where each university has an important Institute of Psychology

with all the research facilities normally found there, we ought to recognize, as Pieron has clearly shown fifteen years ago at the fiftieth anniversary of the *Société française de Psychologie*, that French psychology has only been able to develop in the fringe of official institutions and in constant struggle with the powers that be of academic philosophy. Despite the present progress of the subject, France is still today, by comparison with other countries, one where philosophical studies play the largest part in education (from the twofold point of view of institutions and of intellectual training) and where opportunities for psychological studies have not been very great.

There is certainly a *licence* in psychology of recent date, and which as a result of the psychologist's efforts straddles the two Faculties of Letters and Science (something that philosophical studies should do, as has been the case in Holland as a result of my late friend the logician Beth's initiative). But practically this *licence* leads to very little, for from the point of view of a teaching career there is no *agrégation* in psychology, and from the point of view of a practical career it remains insufficient without the Diplomas of the Institute of Psychology, originating in the no-man's land between official chairs and not having the same official status as the Faculties. Only a few of the provincial Faculties have successfully organized teaching in the subject (Aix-Marseilles and Lille in particular), as this in large measure depends on the interests of the professor of philosophy: both Rennes and Montpellier, where Bourdon and Foucoult have respectively been professors, have been research centers, of which the former alone exists.

The reasons for this situation are clear, although complex. On the one hand, France is the country in which the teaching of philosophy at the level of the *baccalauréat* (the famous "class of philosophy") is the most developed, because it has responded, without referring to the present state of affairs, to a very profound social and vital need for the coordination of values, particularly from the earliest period of secular teaching. The *Célèbres leçons* of J. Lagneau and the fame of Alain's teaching are unambiguous signs of the moral significance of the class of philosophy. This has led public opinion or the collective consciousness to give everything concerning philosophical studies an aura of prestige and authority; and there is thus formed a kind of social élite of philosophers who have the advantage not only of a safe career, but above all of that permanent esteem that plays such a large part in social and administrative decisions at all levels. On the other hand, and this is not due to philosophy, France as a country is not only the most centralized, but also one in which the intellectual gerontocracy successfully holds sway. Thus there is the regimen of competitive examinations with the possibility of imposing syllabuses; the agrégation system, which almost everyone finds absurd (this above all a test of verbal expression) but which one is careful not to change because it gives The Elders a considerable power; the role of "patrons" in the success of a career; the surprising entrenchment of intellectual conservatism that the Institut represents; the custom according to which a retiring professor concerns himself with the succession; all these factors and many others ensure in the main a surprising continuity of doctrine, and in the particular case, give to philosophers the possibility of intellectual and concrete action which they have nowhere else in the education of the younger generation.

In such a sociological context (it is not for nothing that Durkheim's doctrine originated in France!), philosophy remains at the level of an individual or collective wisdom: its permanent tendency to consider itself as a form of knowledge, and more precisely as the highest kind of knowledge, is reinforced in all sorts of ways. For him who has been subjected to philosophy from an early age the question does not even arise, and the student beginning his university studies with the most eminent teachers in the subject has the conviction that an initiation into philosophy allows one to speak of everything. We thus find students becoming specialists in synthesis before all analysis, or entering straightaway into the transcendental world with greater ease as they completely neglect the empirical. And in the only field where they would be able to learn with relative ease what experimental verification is, they prefer the psychology of Sartre and of Merleau-Ponty, where all verification is replaced by arbitrary fiats, to scientific psychology, laborious and appearing alien to the main problems of philosophy.

If I come back to psychology it is not to concern myself with it, since this work is concerned with philosophy, but in order to show how a certain conviction in the powers of general knowledge that philosophy would allow, actually resulted in systematically delaying the rise of an experimental discipline concerned with the mind, and, what is still more significant, dealing with problems of which philosophers have always spoken (for a very large number of them *before* the existence of our science, and for many others who have written afterward, neglecting it more or less deliberately). Among these are nature of perception (which is not a copy but a structuring), the respective roles of experience and the activities of the subject in the formation of concepts, the nature of intellectual operations and of natural logico-mathematical structures, the schematism of memory, decision theory, symbolic function and language, etc. I made these bitter reflections during a meeting of the philosophy section where we had with a good deal of difficulty established (at last!) a chair of experimental psychology and appointed to it the only and excellent candidate present, my friend Paul Fraisse, who specializes, however, in problems of time, in which no metaphysician is disinterested.

Briefly, the implicit permanent principles of the French university authorities are that psychology is part of philosophy, that every philosopher is fit to teach psychology, but that the converse is not true; that there is no question of an *agrégation* in psychology, since the *agrégés* in philosophy know everything; and that experimental inquiry is carried out where it can be, to the extent to which those interested want to concern themselves with it. As a result, for example, during more than fifty years (up to the appointment of Fraisse, who has at last been given the opportunity), the psychological laboratory of the Sorbonne was a peripheral institution, without relationship to the Faculties in spite of the distinguished work carried out there: Binet was not a professor, Pieron was at the Collège de France. Neither Pieron nor Wallon have been members of the Institut, etc.

It has therefore for long been necessary, and it is still partly true, to have a certain amount of heroism in order to study psychology in France, when one is twenty and not a future medical man or engaged in practical affairs. At an age when one is intellectually creative, where it ought to be possible to have the most complete intellectual freedom, one is forced to take part in competitive examinations and to suffer the frightful coercion of the agrégation in philosophy's syllabus.[9] After which one passes for a traitor, humbling oneself performing minor tasks, and proceeding through life at the mercy of events, with a minimum of protection and without any guaranty of having a satisfactory career. The situation has happily improved recently with the creation of an independent section of psychology at the Centre national de la recherche scientifique, but the posts in general depended till now on the philosophy section, then on a joint section with sociology.

(F) I now come to the last part of my account of the experiences of a former future ex-philosopher, which I greatly value, for it has enabled me to make possible a scientific epistemology, such as I have always dreamed of. We need to remember that the boundary between philosophy and science is always changing because it does not depend on the problems themselves, none of which can ever be said to be definitely scientific or metaphysical, but only on their possible delimitation and on the selection of methods enabling us to deal with these circumscribed questions in relying on experimentation, on logico-mathematical formalization or both. I had therefore dreamed of a "genetic epistemology," which would delimit the problems

9 At the Faculty, stress was laid on the excellence of the agrégé of a candidate for such or such a chair, which is of no importance, since it is only a title of a second degree. I thought for my part that I would certainly have failed this great test, being unable to work to a syllabus, and I remembered with pride my little doctorate on the alpine mollusks.

of knowledge in dealing with the question "how does knowledge grow?" which concerns both its formation and historical development. But the criterion of the success of a scientific discipline is intellectual cooperation, and since my disenchantment with philosophy, I have been increasingly of the opinion that any individual piece of work was vitiated by a latent defect, and that to the extent to which one would be able to speak of "Piaget's system," this would be a conclusive proof of my failure.

I had continued on the fringe of psychology, giving courses on genetic epistemology at the Sorbonne and the Faculty of Science of Geneva, but with growing awareness of my limitations, for in order to engage in such a discipline it is not enough to be a psychologist, to have some knowledge of contemporary philosophy, and to be something of a biologist: it is necessary to be a logician, mathematician, physicist, cybernetician, and historian of science, to speak only of the most important. I had published a *Traité de Logique* (very badly named, but this was due to the publisher), but dealing with the development of structures and whose reception by logicians had once again given me the impression of being seated on two or even four stools. I needed therefore to obtain help.

If genetic epistemology is possible, it ought also to be necessarily interdisciplinary. Holding this conviction strongly, I tried to prove it and sent a program of research to the Rockefeller Foundation. J. Marshall, who was friendly toward me, at first replied that his colleagues, whom he had consulted, had found nothing in it that differed from ongoing research in the U.S.A. I replied by proposing that an Anglo-Saxon epistemologist spend three months at Geneva and make a report to the Foundation as to whether our results agreed with or differed from American and English studies. The Foundation agreed to this and W. Mays of Manchester came to Geneva, where he has written a very intelligent report, which enabled my project to go forward. But as my ambitious project interested all departments, I have been subjected to the customary tests, consisting in one or two excellent dinners on the top story of the Rockefeller Building in New York, in the company of the heads of these departments who had prepared their examination questions. These questions were almost all of a surprising pertinence. I remember the practical questions: How will you find people sufficiently intelligent so as to achieve a real collaboration and at the same time sufficiently stupid to abandon for a year their studies in mathematics or logic, etc., and to embark on a dialogue with "child psychologists"? But I particularly remember the theoretical questions, due among others to Weaver, the mathematician interested in information theory who was then in charge of the Department of Science at the Foundation: How will you find interesting epistemological ideas, for example, the theory of relativity, in studying children who know nothing and who in any case are brought up in the intellectual tradition dating from Newton? What do children think of set-theory and of the one-to-one correspondence used by Cantor, *et al.*? I had the luck to be able to remark on the first point that Einstein himself had advised me in 1928 to study the formation of the intuitions of velocity in order to see if they depended on those of duration, and that further, when I had the good fortune to see Einstein again at Princeton (I stayed three months at the Oppenheimer Institute, where he was permanently resident), he was quite delighted by the reactions of nonconservation of children of four to six years (they deny that a liquid conserves its quantity when it is poured from one glass into another of a different shape: "There is more to drink than before," etc.), and was greatly astonished that the elementary concepts of conservation were only constructed toward seven or eight years. As for the second question, I was able to answer Weaver that children readily handle one-to-one correspondence, and that the study of this problem shows that the transition from logical class to number in the child is much more complex than the formal account of this relationship given by Whitehead and Russell in *Principia Mathematica*. In short, I tried to cope with them, and some months later obtained the necessary funds for establishing a "*Centre international d'Épistémologie génétique*" in the Faculty of Science of Geneva.

The beginnings were not easy. In order to make a team of Geneva psychologists work with two logicians and one mathematician, we had to begin by finding a common language and a good few months were required before we came to understand each other, especially the logicians and psychologists. The mathematician was neither as intelligent nor as stupid as the Rockefeller administrator had imagined in his pessimistic predictions: he came to Geneva but in order to continue his own work in a peaceful setting, and, if he gave us some good ideas, he disinterested himself tolerably well from the fortunes of genetic epistemology, except at the final symposium, where he was very active. (I have learned since then that this disinterest outside his own work was not directed at our growing Center, but was a permanent feature of his method of working.) However, the work of the Center went on tolerably dealing with such topics as "logic and equilibrium," the relations between logic and language, etc., when during the year W. Mays suggested that we test experimentally the famous problem of synthetic and analytic relations, a central problem for the school of logical empiricism and which had put at odds supporters of that school with the well-known Harvard logician Quine. I had invited to the Center for this first year the Belgian logician Apostel so as to compare our views with those of a supporter of logical positivism, a doctrine in which he still believed, and to see if the facts would arbitrate between our respective views opposed on essential points: the exclusive role of experience or the structuring activity of the subject, etc. We started our work with zeal, Apostel, Mays, Morf, and myself, the first being inclined to believe that we would find from childhood a sharp opposition between synthetic or empirical judgments and analytic or logico-mathematical ones, the last being of the opinion that we would find all intermediaries and all combinations.

This was an interesting experiment, at first because it questioned that which Quine has called one of the "dogmas" of logical empiricism, and then because it was for us the first time that two epistemologists equally convinced of their respective theses, but which were contradictory, proceeded to test them against the same facts. I was, however, convinced that there was no such thing as a pure fact, but that, as Duhem, Poincaré, and so many others have shown, it always involves an interpretation (which, nevertheless, is in itself a refutation of positivism or logical empiricism). Would we therefore be able to agree on the interpretations? Such was the importance for me of the stake of this first experiment in real collaboration. The facts seemed to me to establish my point: alongside clearly synthetic physical relationships and clearly analytic logical ones (the criterion being simply whether the subject finds it necessary to make use of verification in order to come to a decision), we found relationships which were logico-mathematical and at the same time synthetic: for example, that five counters in a row no longer make five when the row is split up into two of $3 + 2$ elements and that the relationship $5 = 3 + 2$ only becomes necessary after a construction (itself being an integral part of a "group"), etc. Apostel was, however, far from agreeing and with admirable subtlety multiplied the possible interpretations between physical numbering, insofar as the names of numbers are only used for measurement, and mathematical numbering. We therefore had to embark on the task of defining concepts and formulating criteria and in applying them to the collected facts, and no less than three successive drafts were needed, each copiously amended by the other author, before we were able to conclude. This study has appeared [10] and it was clear from it that if there was not complete agreement it was almost complete: Apostel admitted the existence of intermediaries between the analytic and synthetic, but believed in a genetic dependency leading from physical relationships to logico-mathematical ones (two theses in the end contrary to logical empiricism at least in its orthodox form), while I maintained the distinction at all ages

[10] L. Apostel, W. Mays, A. Morf, and J. Piaget, *Les liaisons analytiques et synthétiques dans les comportements du sujet*, "Etudes d'épistémologie génétique," Vol. IV, Paris, Presses Universitaires de France.

of the physical and the logico-mathematical, but believed in all the transitions between the synthetic and analytic.

The experiment was therefore convincing: an honest examination of the facts, combined with an elaboration in part formalized of the interpretations, can lead epistemologists initially in disagreement with each other to revise and state more precisely their hypotheses so as to come close to agreement, in any case much superior to the conflicting positions started from. We now had to wait for the reaction of others. W. V. Quine had declined with understandable discretion, when the Center was first founded, to be a member of its Advisory Board. When he read the volume on *L'analytique et le synthétique* (whose Introduction, due to Apostel, showed clearly by bringing together the many theses of contemporary philosophers that the question is constantly stated in terms of facts and not only of pure logic), he wrote us a very encouraging letter, recognizing the scope of the collected facts, while making reservations as to the mode of definition adopted, and accepting retrospectively membership on the Board of the Center.

We had, on the other hand, to face the ten distinguished guests whom we had invited (as was the case in all later years) to a final symposium in order to discuss the studies completed during the year and to prepare those for the following year. We had invited E. W. Beth, F. Gonseth, A. Naess, J. Bruner, etc., a group of logicians, mathematicians, psychologists, all interested in epistemology, and we had no clear idea what the discussion simply of our own studies by specialists, whom we had not asked to give a lecture or a personal paper, would produce over the period of one week.

I was particularly concerned about one of the guests, the logician Beth of Amsterdam, who had published in *Methodos* at Father Bochenski's request a savage review of my *Traité de logique*. I have written a reply of several pages, which Father Bochenski simply refused to publish (no purpose will be served in stressing this conception of philosophical objectivity). But he allowed me several lines and I limited myself to saying that I

understood extremely well that a pure logician would be highly
critical of an attempt to formalize certain structures selected
because they belonged to natural thought, but that there is a
problem here and the only way of understanding each other
would be for us to publish a joint work on such topics, in which
neither the logician nor the psychologist would by himself be
adequate for the task. I have written at length to Beth in the
same vein proposing that we put our respective interests on one
side and seriously undertake this work. Beth, who was a very
honest man, said he was surprised and touched by this request
and has not declined the proposed collaboration, but asked to
be allowed to think about it. I was therefore somewhat anxious
as to what he would think and say at the symposium.

The latter gave us complete satisfaction. From the first ses-
sion Beth found the demonstration, by unexpected topological
considerations, of a proposition that Apostel was trying to justify
in the field of the relations between language, logic, and information (and codes minimizing error). Arne Naess, who works
in the field of the experimental epistemology of adults, if one
may put it thus, at Oslo, was full of helpful remarks, particularly
on analytic and synthetic relationships, and stressed the importance of the genetic dimension in connection with adults. My
old friend Gonseth, for whom the philosophy of science is essentially "open," opened his mind to all our concerns. The discussions were really "working sessions" and not uncoordinated im-
provisations as in so many congresses (a maximum of ten guests
is an absolute limit here). At the end of this symposium I had
the impression that genetic epistemology existed, and what was
more encouraging, Beth had it too.[11]

[11] Our projected collaboration resulted in a volume: *Epistémologie
mathématique et psychologie*, Vol. XIX of the *Etudes d'épistémologie
génétique*, Presses Universitaires de France, 1961. (*Mathematical Epistemology and Psychology*. Translation and foreword by W. Mays, D. Reidel,
1966). Without resulting in a detailed collaboration because of the geo-
graphical distance separating us, each drafted his part, which was carefully
revised by the other, and Beth himself drafted the main points of the general conclusions held in common, which satisfied me completely with re-

The Center continued its work for seven years with the help of the Rockefeller Foundation; when the latter ceased to subsidize us its financing was taken over by the *Fonds national suisse de la Recherche scientifique*. The results of this work, which have appeared in about twenty volumes in the collection *Etudes d'épistémologie génétique*, Presses Universitaires de France, have dealt with the formation, learning, and genealogy of logical structures, the "reading off" of experience, the problems of number and space, the concepts of function, time, velocity, and causality, and we are thinking of studying the problems of biological epistemology.

It is important to note, from the point of view of those of us who wish to make epistemology into a science, that these results have been due above all to a continual interdisciplinary collaboration, without anyone among us ever having had the impression of being self-sufficient. This cooperation, established on a weak level from the first year, has only become stronger, and in this respect it can be said that the Center has succeeded. The credit for this is, of course, due to the excellent collaborators, all of whom I cannot name, but I should like to mention some of them.

Pierre Gréco came out first several years ago in the *agrégation* in philosophy (this was not the reason for my choice), was my assistant at the Sorbonne, then my Director of Research, and later obtained leave of absence in order to work at the Center: he specialized in genetic psychology, but was concerned as much as I am with epistemological problems, for which his training as a *normalien* gave him a wide knowledge. He has carried out excellent investigations on number, the learning of logical structures, space, time, and causality, and has shown in each of them a surprising aptitude for experimental programming and verification.

J. B. Grize is a logician who, before going to study with the Belgian logicians, had defended a thesis on the elimination of

gard to the necessary epistemological collaboration between logicians and psychologists.

time in the history of mathematical concepts. Although both a logician and a mathematician (he teaches at present in the Faculty of Letters of Neuchâtel and of Science of Geneva), this has not prevented him, no doubt due to his historical interests, from adapting himself immediately and intimately to genetic questions. He has worked, of major importance to us, in the formalization of the natural structures of the different levels of development and in particular formalized my ideas on the construction of number.

L. Apostel is another logician, brought up in the logical positivist tradition, but very open to genetic questions as to a variety of others. His surprising energy showed itself both by a constant fertility of ideas and by an increasingly personal approach having regard to his initial tendencies.

S. Papert has two doctorates in mathematics (one from Cambridge on the foundations of topology), had worked at the *Institut Poincaré* and on cybernetics at the National Physical Laboratory, London. Fundamentally polyvalent, he also concerned himself when at Johannesburg (with Taylor) with experiments on perception by means of distorting spectacles. His polyvalence had convinced him of the existence of the subject, and his epistemology is centered on the constructions of this subject, expressed in turn in terms of psychology, logic (Papert was nearly appointed to a senior post in logic at Cambridge), and cybernetic programming, without forgetting his very lively neurological interests. Papert was therefore the ideal collaborator for the Center, whose ideas he enthusiastically defended and enriched, and has produced a large number of studies, beginning with a criticism of reductionist logic, continuing with a cybernetic model of development or the "genetron" (which is able to pass through levels of equilibrium as in real development, instead of proceeding by an equilibrium starting again at zero in the case of failure, therefore by all or none, as in Ashby's homeostat), then with researches on functions and time.

We have been much helped by others in a series of special problems: F. Bresson, who concerned himself with perceptual schematism and causality, had a remarkable feeling for abstract and concrete "models"; G. Th. Guilbaud, whose inexhaustible erudition has thrown light on many questions, among others explanation in mathematics; C. Nowinski, versed in dialectic and Polish logic; Gruber of New York, who works in perception and biological epistemology; F. Meyer of Aix-en-Provence, whose fine book *La problématique de l'évolution* has much impressed us, etc. At the annual symposia we have had the privilege of the collaboration of W. V. Quine, the Harvard logician, W. McCulloch, the distinguished co-originator of the "logic of neurons," the physicists Halbwachs, D. Rivier, and O. Costa de Beauregard, of G.-G. Granger, the epistemologist of the human sciences, without referring to former collaborators who have become regulars at these meetings, in particular L. Apostel.

The activities of the *Centre d'épistémologie génétique* have aroused the interest of our colleagues in the Faculty of Science, who have seen the possible value of such studies for the theory of scientific thought; among others the mathematician G. de Rham and the biologist F. Chodat. The new generation of philosophers of the Faculty of Letters has, on the contrary, shown a distrust which I took to be a symptom of the effects of phenomenology, and I have compared this generation knowing nothing of science with that of Reymond, Brunschvicg, and Lalande, who were, however, philosophers in spirit. Jeanne Hersch has never spoken to me about epistemology, but asked me one day: "Do you believe that psychology is a science? I must explain to you . . ." I fear that I let her see my intense internal amusement, for I have never received the explanation: on the other hand, we shall soon see what this led to. R. Schaerer's interest in our subject, as that of almost all the present members of the *Société romande de Philosophie* (which has asked Grize to give an account of our methods), is to praise our child studies, but to point out that they have no significance as far as the adult is concerned, nor above all for knowledge. R. Schaerer has given some thought to this subject in a discussion of the *Recontres internationales*, and in Chapter Five I will examine the value of his arguments. But the intentions of J. Hersch and of R. Scha-erer can be quite clearly seen from a project whose full import will be appreciated, *viz* to teach philosophical psychology in the Faculty of Letters so as to complete psychology as under-stood in science, and to entrust this teaching to F. Mueller, whose *Histoire de la psychologie* (which exhibits, following philosophical usage, a better knowledge of texts than of facts) concluded that scientific psychology is unable to give us the "philosophical anthropology" that we need. After unanimous protests from the psychologists, the Faculty of Letters has de-cided to rename the chair "History of Philosophical Psychol-ogy," and this is real progress, for it may well be that such a discipline already belongs to history. It is true that we know nothing of this and that we ought to refrain from making any prediction. But if I am right and if, moreover, genetic episte-mology has some future, it is worth noting that at the moment when our Center prepared this future, the philosophers of the Faculty of Letters of Geneva were concerned with reviving phil-osophical psychology. It is on this note of pride that I end the account of my disenchantment and this lengthy confession, which tells of my subjective illusions, is certainly sincere.

Science
and Philosophy

PHILOSOPHY takes up a rational position to the whole of reality. We use the term "rational" to contrast philosophy with purely practical or affective positions or again with beliefs simply accepted without a reflective elaboration: a pure morality, a faith, etc. The concept "the whole of reality" involves three components. Firstly, it refers to the whole of the higher activities of man and not exclusively to knowledge: moral, aesthetic, faith (religious or humanist), etc. Secondly, from the point of view of knowledge, it implies the possibility that, underlying phenomenal appearance and individual knowledge, there exists an ultimate reality, a thing in itself, an absolute, etc. Thirdly, that a reflection on the whole of reality can give an insight into the realm of possibility (Leibniz, Renouvier, etc.).

(A) For some philosophies the thing in itself exists, but is unknowable; this position is in this respect then based on practical reason. Nonetheless these philosophies are concerned with the whole of reality. Other philosophies, like dialectical materialism, appear to limit reality to the perceived or spatiotemporal universe. But the term "materialism" means in fact belief in the existence of objects, independently of the subject: an object is thus often taken by the "materialist" as a limit in the mathematical sense, approached by successive approximations without it ever being reached. On the other hand, if dialectical materialism attacks idealism, it constantly stresses action, or *praxis*, from a social point of view, as well as the role of action in the case of individual knowledge. (Marx, for example, already showed himself critical of Feuerbach's sensationalism by arguing that perception is based on an "activity" of man's senses.) It is therefore clear that dialectical materialism also comes within the proposed definition, with this important difference, that a dialectical approach is substituted for a static one, but one having all the features of a rational approach to the whole of reality, the concept of totality being central to Marxism.

Only one philosophy accepts a more limited position in relation to our definition, although coming within it again formally. This is positivism, not that of Comte, which banishes metaphysics in order to replace it by a "subjective synthesis," but contemporary "logical positivism," which reduces the whole of reality to physical phenomena and a language. This once again is a conception like any other of "the whole of reality," and as this position is a highly "rational" one, it therefore comes within the terms of a definition endeavoring to cover all systems. In what follows we will be able to set aside such a position as its avowed aim is to limit the number of *problems* and not only to specify methods. We ought, in fact, to make three important reservations in respect of such a doctrine, which Oppenheimer one day called a "humorless philosophy."

Firstly, and from the point of view of science itself, the latter cannot be limited to a group of problems considered in themselves alone as "scientific." Contemporary science is essentially "open" and remains free to include any new problems that it wishes or is able to, as long as it can find methods for dealing with them. In the physical field one has vainly tried to banish causality and to insist that it be subject to law; nevertheless the search for a causal explanation remains more than ever an essential need of the mind. In the psychological field one has tried to exclude "mentalism" and Bloomfield has asserted that to look for "concepts" under the syntagmas of language is only a matter for theologians and literary men; Soviet psychology nonetheless concerns itself with the problem of consciousness and the internalization of actions into thought still remains the central psychological problem of the cognitive functions.

Secondly, to assert that metaphysical problems are "meaningless" is unacceptable from the point of view of knowledge itself, not that the validity of metaphysical knowledge can be accepted without question (which we will question ourselves later on), but because we are not justified in definitely classifying a problem as either scientific or metaphysical; at the most a disputed problem can be said to be "without present (cognitive) meaning." The question whether below the microscopic level, physical reality exhibits an underlying determinism or a basic indeterminism would have been generally classified as "metaphysical" at the end of the last century. It is nonetheless a present-day problem in physics, one which L. de Broglie opposes to the position of the Copenhagen school. As for the problem of human freedom, it has by now been stripped of all scientific meaning, since any technique of verification only allows us to decide either for or against one of the proposed solutions and in such a field the evidence of the inner self is particularly suspect of partiality. Nevertheless, we discover that by an extension of Gödel's theorem on the impossibility of demonstrating the non-contradiction of a system (sufficiently rich) by its own methods or by weaker methods, contemporary cybernetics raises the problem of determinism in limited but precise terms. A machine sufficiently complex to simulate an intellectual task, and rigorously determined as far as its mechanism and its interactions with the external world, cannot compute at a time t what its state will be at a time $t + 1$; it can only do this to the extent to which its determination, incomplete in itself, is subordinated to a machine of a higher order, but which is then no longer completely self-determined; and so on. We see once again that a problem without present meaning can suddenly acquire one as a result of advances in thought that were unforeseen.

Thirdly, and I want to emphasize this strongly so as to avoid all misunderstanding, a problem not having a present meaning from the cognitive point of view is nonetheless, in many cases, a problem having a permanent human meaning and is consequently a legitimate philosophical problem. As an example, let us take what is undoubtedly the most central problem motivating all philosophy: that of the meaning of life, often called the problem of the "finality" of existence. To begin with finality, this concept is the prototype of those concepts that positivism considers to be metaphysical and nonscientific, and rightly so, since it concerns an anthropocentric idea, originating in a confusion between conscious subjective data and the causal mechanism of action, and involving, under the form of "final causes," a determination of the present by the future. However, this illusory concept covers objective relations of functional value, adaptation, anticipatory regulation, etc., of such a sort that the problem remains and has given rise in the field of cybernetics to solutions often termed "mechanical equivalents of finality": such are systems having loops or *feedbacks* and with recent progress *feedforwards* or regulations of the second degree. Thus we have today a scientific concept, and no longer a metaphysical one, corresponding to finality (which positivism would never have foreseen, since by limiting scientific problems, it would never have made such hypotheses). This concept is made the basis of studies called "teleonomy," which, it has been facetiously said, is related to teleology as astronomy is to astrology. Does the problem of the meaning or the finality of life have a present cognitive meaning, and in particular can it be related to the concepts of teleonomy? Clearly not; to give an intellectual or cognitive expression to the concept of the finality of life is to make it either the result of a pre-established plan of divine order, or the locus of an immanent finality, of a progressive development, etc. These are, however, hypotheses, let us not say undemonstrable (we know nothing about this) but undemonstrated, since they do not convince everyone, and to call them "metaphysical truths" is another way of saying that they are not truths pure and simple, therefore not truths in the full sense of the word. Let us therefore grant to the positivist that such a problem is without (present) meaning from the cognitive point of view. But nonetheless, without reference to the possibility of verification, this problem remains central from the point of view of human existence and the thinking subject, for we have a choice between a life without values, a life with relative and unstable values, and a life involving values experienced as absolute, engaging one's whole being. To deny such a problem because it is a vital one and without positive cognitive solutions is plainly absurd, since it constantly occurs and forces itself on us in the form of "engagement," even if we do not know how to formulate it intellectually. And it is the same with a large number of problems.

The essential characteristic of a complete man is without a doubt to refuse to confuse generic distinctions and to accept as demonstrated truths what are only hypotheses. But it is also to refuse to compartmentalize or to fragment his personality, such that on the one hand, he limits himself to observing, reasoning and verifying, and on the other, to remain content with believing in values that engage and direct him, without his being able to understand them. On the contrary, a thinking subject in possession of knowledge and values, necessarily tries to construct a general conception that will bring them under one form or another; such is the role of philosophy insofar as it is a rational approach to the whole of reality. Every thinking man adopts or makes for himself a philosophy, even if his general conception and his understanding of values remains for him approximate and personal. We need then to discover why philosophy has become a specialized discipline and what this means.

(B) A philosophical position involves a general conception concerned, among other things, with knowledge. This provides a twofold reason why it tends to be regarded as a form of knowledge. But this way of speaking is only relative to modern man, for whom there exists a more or less clear-cut difference between science and philosophy and, in some fields, as in the exact sciences, a very sharp distinction.

The most important reason, which is a historical one, why philosophy has always been considered as a form of knowledge in our Western civilization, is that it has long been bound up with science, from the time of the earliest Greek thinkers, for whom the distinction between science and philosophy did not exist. When the pre-Socratics began to think about reality in a rational manner and no longer in the symbolic language of the myth, their conceptions of the world involved at one and the same time philosophy and physics as in the case of the school of Miletus, or mathematics as in the case of Pythagoreanism, or cosmology, etc. For our purpose it is important to note how this connection with science has remained alive for so long. But before going on to this, we also need to note that this is a characteristic of Western rather than Oriental thought. It is clearly not accidental that Oriental philosophy sees itself much more than ours does as being essentially a wisdom, whereas a lesser development of science and technology would have allowed us to avoid a too systematic polarization of values on to the field of knowledge.

The initial interdependence of philosophy and science is generally presented as if the former had at first "included" the latter, which then has gradually become separated from it. This is not false if we give a static description of the stages of this development, which are then related together in a serial fashion. But the important problem is to discover the reason for the succession of systems: granting that the coordination of values is the permanent function of philosophy, and that the terms of the problem vary relatively little in relation to the evolution of knowledge. The question is, as far as the latter is concerned, whether it is a progress toward this complete knowledge, the goal of philosophy, which has led to the particular kinds of knowledge becoming separated from the common matrix in the form of specialized sciences; or whether, on the contrary, it is progress of a scientific nature (inside or outside the field termed philosophical, this does not matter), which, by forcing us to reflect anew on the knowledge thus transformed, has brought about the development of systems.

In saying that it does not matter if scientific progress which, on the second hypothesis, would have involved philosophical reflection, is due to a thinker referred to today as a mathematician, etc., or to someone else who is classed today among the philosophers, I lay myself open to the reply that, in the second case at least, it is philosophers who have led the movement. It is of no help to say that science and philosophy were at first undifferentiated, since we are looking for the factor that led to this progress: either the application of this complete knowledge (or the search for it) to the results of the specialized kinds of knowledge, or, on the contrary, research in the latter which has produced new effort of reflective analysis, leading to the construction of general systems. We need to recall that there is no difference in nature between philosophical and scientific cognitive problems. They only differ in their delimitation or specialization and above all in their methods, which are either purely reflective or based upon systematic or experimental observation in the case of facts and rigorous algorithms in the case of deduction. It is therefore relatively easy, or at least possible, to know broadly on which matters a philosopher has engaged in scientific activity or to which he has tended to have a scientific attitude (since this is primarily a matter of approach and not of boundaries in the static sense), and those about which he only philosophizes. Two examples will suffice.

When Aristotle directed the work of his three hundred assistants in order to obtain the data necessary for his biology, and discovered such facts as that the Cetacea are mammals and not fish, etc., there is little doubt that he engaged in scientific activity. Even if Aristotle had been guided by more general reflections (which is undoubtedly the case with all innovators), he was not content to extend them by solitary meditation and went on to study the facts in collaboration with others. When, on the other hand, he constructs his system, his ideas on potentiality and actuality, his general interpretation of forms as immanent in reality and no longer in the world of Ideas, he is certainly a philosopher. It is therefore not unreasonable to assume that it is the biological interests of Aristotle and the mathematical interests of Plato that account for the essential differences in their systems, and this is commonplace. On the other hand, we need to ask whether these great innovators have not been great precisely because they have based themselves on *results*, either logico-mathematical or due to methodological observation, and not *only* on ideas, however necessary the latter may be. Comparing them with Plotinus,[1] who still believed that mountains grew like giant mushrooms, we find a slight difference, and it is this which our teaching programs neglect when they assume that philosophers can be produced by the dozen, without their first having a scientific training.

Descartes, who lived at a time when science and philosophy were already differentiated, is the best example to quote, not because he is superior to Leibniz, whose position was the same from the point of view which concerns us here, but because he explained very clearly the working relationship which he established between his philosophical and scientific activities. One needs, he said, to spend only one day a month on philosophy (something again neglected by our teaching programs) and to spend the others in tasks such as computation or dissection. If Descartes has discovered analytical geometry, enabling him to coordinate numerical and spatial quantities, is it because of his general doctrine of thought and extension, two substances which he had so much difficulty in considering at one and the same time as distinct and inseparably united, or can one assume that the studies with which he was concerned twenty-nine or thirty days of each month, have had some influence on the conceptions elaborated during the remaining day?

(C) If one accepts these methodological points, it seems undeniable that the most important systems in the history of philosophy, that is to say those which have given rise to others and which have themselves had a lasting influence, have all arisen from a reflection on the scientific discoveries of their authors themselves or on a scientific revolution occurring in a period in which they lived or immediately preceding it. Thus

---

[1] Without wishing to lessen the interest of Plotinus for religious philosophy, in a field where rightly the coordination of values prevails over the cognitive meaning.

Plato was concerned with mathematics, Aristotle with logic and biology, Descartes with algebra and analytical geometry, Leibniz with the infinitesimal calculus, the empiricists Locke and Hume with their studies anticipatory of psychology, Kant with Newtonian science and its generalizations, Hegel and Marx with history and sociology, and Husserl with Frege's logistic. And let us again note by way of a counterproof, that systems that have had no connections with science have not been successful in producing an original epistemology and have rather stressed the defense and interpretation of values, in the form of a transcendental theology in Plotinus' case, a rigorously immanent one in that of Spinoza, or in a radical idealism as in the German post-Kantians.

Starting from this epistemological point of view, which is that in which philosophy comes closest to knowledge in the strict sense, it is of some interest to note that the great philosophical systems owe to the kind of science which has given them their epistemological orientation, not only the emphasis put on this epistemology but also the particular kinds of epistemology that they have adopted, which is more instructive. We will in this respect distinguish six kinds.

1. First there is Platonic realism, which projects the structures of knowledge into a suprasensible world without their depending on either a human or transcendental subject. The subject is therefore not active in knowledge and is limited, by reminiscence or participation, to the reflection of the eternal Ideas, the latter, moreover, forming the basis for the supreme values, moral, aesthetic, and religious. This realism of transcendent Ideas was the only epistemology compatible with the peculiar status of Greek mathematics. Although it had had a rational and operational character from the time of Pythagoras, it put all the stress, in virtue of the known psychological laws, on the result of these operations and not on their functioning, for conscious realization starts from the peripheral result of actions before turning to their inner mechanism, which, more-

E

over, it never completely attains. From this resulted a systematic and essentially static realism, which made Pythagoras believe that numbers were in things, in the manner of spatial atoms. The important consequences of this belief were: Euclid's opposition to using motion, reluctance in handling the infinite, difficulties in the analysis of the continuum, the rejection of the so-called mechanical curves, which were thought of as due to human artifice and not as belonging to reality in the same way as the geometrical figures obtained by rule and compass alone; scruples about algebra, conceived of as a simple procedure of computation and not as a science with the same status as geometry. And finally, the inability to construct a dynamic mathematical physics for lack of an operational treatment of motion and time (cf. Zeno) and even the concept of a directional time. Such a systematic and static realism could not remain tied to the perceived world, and it has become separated from it from the time of the crisis produced within Pythagoreanism by the discovery of irrationals: if there are mathematical entities irreducible to a simple relationship between two integers, it is because number, while being external to us, is not "in" the things. Plato's genius consisted in separating out the epistemology implicit in this general situation. We thus see that, if the pre-Socratics concerned themselves with activities that could be described as scientific or pre-scientific as well as philosophical, the first of the great philosophies of Western civilization originated from reflection upon an already constituted science.

2. Aristotle was not a mathematician but he has both founded logic and developed biology. In these two fields he has found "forms" that recall the Platonic Forms or Ideas, but in one case embodied in the subject's discourse and in the other in the structure of the organism. If he had been conscious of the activities of the epistemological or operational subject, and not merely of the individual subject,[2] through his perceptions

[2] We do not, of course, oppose epistemological and individual in the sense of the opposition between transcendental and psychological: both of them arise from psychology as from epistemology. The epistemological sub-

and sensory organs, and if he had had some intuition of the evolution of the species as had so clearly this new Aristotle, which Leibniz was, he would without a doubt have produced a theory of the progressive construction of logical forms starting from organic forms. But he accepted the same systematic and static realism as did Plato and the whole of Greek thought, while reintroducing the forms into physical or spatio-temporal reality according to a second kind of epistemology, which we might call immanent realism. Greek thought has, in fact, remained alien to the concept of an active epistemological subject, and the only two powers that Aristotle attributed to the subject are those of a conscious realization of forms and an abstraction starting from perceptions enabling a content to be given to the forms. To be sure, the Sophists, rehabilitated by Dupréel, have stressed the need for a certain norm of subjectivity, but their aim seemed above all to be critical and they did not arrive at the epistemological subject. When Protagoras declared that man is the measure of all things, either he did not go beyond the individual subject, as Plato interpreted it, or he glimpsed an epistemological relativism still far removed from the idea of construction. As for the idea of evolution, it was even further away from Greek thought than were the concepts of mathematical and physical transformations, and the universal becoming of Heraclitus does not exhibit time's arrow, since it involves an eternal recurrence which he or his disciples admitted. The theory of forms in Aristotle, instead of being directed toward a dialectical constructivism ended therefore in a static hierarchy, the higher stages of which explained the lower ones, and whose built-in finality and the concept of a passage from potentiality to actuality excluded any epistemology of the subject's activity. It is nevertheless true that this famous doctrine draws upon two kinds of inspiration, which form the starting point of two of the most important sciences of today: logic and biology.

---

ject refers to the general coordination of actions (combining, ordering, etc.) constitutive of logic, and the individual subject to the specific and differentiated actions of each individual taken separately.

3. Descartes' discovery of the epistemological subject as well as the very detail of his philosophy would be inexplicable without three mathematical and physical innovations that have forced him to revise Aristotle's epistemology and to rethink the conditions of knowledge. Firstly, the development of algebra has brought to the fore the possibility of a discipline based on the subject's operations and on their arbitrary combination, and no longer on geometrical figures experienced as external or on numbers considered as existing independently of the operations that engendered them. Secondly, Descartes' discovery of analytical geometry showed him the possibility of an exact correspondence between algebra, the domain of thought operations, and geometry the domain of extension, from which arises the permanent Cartesian theme of the relations between thought and extension, which are at one and the same time indissociable and basically distinct. Thirdly, Galileo's discoveries concerning inertial motion, his fundamental method consisting in taking time, henceforth uni-directional, as an independent variable; and in a general fashion, the possibility of applying computational methods to physical transformations (transformations that have taken on a rational character as a result of the deductive coordination of change and an invariant), are innovations having considerable significance. These explain at one and the same time the Cartesian conception of causality as the logico-mathematical reason for the transformations, the rejection of finality and the rejection (improper) of the idea of force, because Aristotle thought of it as a substantial and nontransitive property of the physical body (theory of the two movers, making the internal mover the equivalent still quasi-animistic of a kind of animal instinct having motor properties).

But if under the influence of these three major events, Descartes discovered by means of logico-mathematical methods the epistemological subject and its power of radically assimilating physical reality, he remained, as was the case with Leibniz, in a position intermediary between the absence of a subject in Plato and Aristotle and the structuring subject of Kantian *a priorism*.

We may describe this third kind of epistemological position as a doctrine of "pre-established harmony," although the phrase is Leibnizian and Leibniz used the concept to explain how the monad, shut in upon itself, nevertheless conceives ideas that correspond to external realities. But Descartes, for whom they were categories constitutive of reason, considered them as innate ideas, and if one does not interpret the correspondence between innate ideas and reality in terms of an *a-priori* structuring, one can only, in a static and nonevolutionary conception of man, refer to a pre-established harmony. The great interest of Descartes' position is that he did not reduce everything to innate ideas and that over and above them and in "adventitious" ideas (of perceptual origin), he recognizes the existence of "factitious" ideas due to mental operations, as is the case with algebraic concepts whose importance in the discovery of the epistemological subject we have noted. We have here, therefore, proof of a historical conscious realization of "operations" (in opposition to Greek thought), and definite evidence that an introspective conscious realization is no substitute for an objective and genetic psychological study. The analysis of the development of logico-mathematical operations in the child in fact shows, on the one hand, that even concepts appearing to be derived from perception involve a much more complex operational structuring than had seemed to be the case, and on the other, that the important categories considered by Descartes as innate are a refined product of this operational structuring.

4. Leibniz's system, like that of Descartes, was, as is well known, directly influenced by his own scientific discoveries. He has derived the principles of continuity and indiscernibles from the infinitesimal calculus, and its applications have led him to the philosophical use which he made of the principle of sufficient reason. Proceeding from the algebra of the finite to that of the infinite, which is his new calculus, he has grasped better than anyone else the dynamic operational character of intelligence and has been able to answer Locke that the latter's empiricism could not explain the *ipse intellectus*. But convinced

of the unrestricted extension of the physical applications made possible by his calculus, he did not accept an idealism, which he might have done if he had only concerned himself with the new powers that he discovered in the activities of the epistemological subject. On the other hand, considering these activities as closed on themselves, which is consistent both with the spirit of mathematical structuralism as well as with logical demonstration, of which he gave the earliest examples and saw its future possibilities (see the excellent studies on his logic by B. Russell and Conturat), but considering, as against this, the close agreement between logico-mathematical knowledge and physical reality, he found a compromise in the hypothesis of monads, whose functioning is closed although corresponding to all the events of the universe. From this follows his pre-established harmony or "perfect parallelism" which simultaneously takes account of experimental knowledge, of the relations between mind and body, and of the intuitive residues discovered even in the most abstract ideas.

5. While the construction of new logico-mathematical structures led Descartes and Leibniz to the discovery of the epistemological subject, psychological considerations gave rise in Great Britain to a fourth kind of epistemological interpretation, to be seen in Locke's empiricism, then in Hume's. The position characteristic of innatism and the hypothesis of a pre-established harmony is, in fact, an unstable one. It assumes that either the subject in general is only the reflection or the locus of structures which exist independently of itself, and there is no epistemological subject as in kinds I and II, or that there is an epistemological subject and it plays an active role in knowledge, in the form of a structuring, which it imposes a priori, on all experience or under the form of a progressive construction conserving the internal necessity characteristic of the a priori, but under a dynamic and no longer static form. To adhere to innate ideas is to limit this construction, either a priori or dialectically, in favor of a kind of pre-formation or predetermination which remains halfway between the initial realism and later achievements.

Because of this empiricism has questioned the hypothesis of innateness, using quite new arguments whose later historical development showed that they formed the starting point of an independent science: psychology founded on methodological observation and experiment. Locke wanted to start from the facts and no longer to resolve questions by metaphysical deduction, and Hume gave to his *Treatise* the subtitle: *being an attempt to introduce the experimental method of reasoning into moral subjects*. While Descartes and Leibniz explicitly admitted the innateness of the basic ideas for deductive reasons, basing themselves essentially on their universality and necessity, the empiricists have had the great merit of looking for verification in the facts, stating the problem in a way glimpsed by Aristotle, but which was new in its generality and its absence from all presuppositions: how are ideas formed in reality, *i.e.* as they appear to observation and experiment? They have, of course, only observed a progressive and in part variable formation, with little sign of the pre-formation implied by the theory of innate ideas. Further, proceeding themselves by an empirical method, they have only observed in the factors constitutive of the origin of ideas the part played by experience with, in addition, an organizing factor that Locke referred to by the global phrase "operations of our mind" known by reflection, and Hume reduced it to the association of ideas.

But if empiricism thus opened the way to a whole group of fundamental and extremely fruitful inquiries, it has itself proceeded somewhat apace, remaining satisfied with a minimum of effort. In fact the kinds of observations and experiments which it was looking for only started in a methodological fashion in the nineteenth century and it is still for most of the important questions at the phase of a first approximation. The empiricists themselves were content to proceed *more philosophico*, *i.e.* reflecting much and appealing to facts by way of examples and justification: in such cases the facts, of course, always confirm the hypotheses. We do not therefore need to refer to empiricist philosophy in order to judge the value of the experimental methods in determining the mechanism of cognitive functions, as do many other writers in an unreflective and sometimes even deliberate fashion. Two very different aspects are to be distinguished in the empiricist movement. On the one hand, the desire to test methodologically our hypotheses against the facts of experience, which was only a pious hope a century or two before there was an experimental discipline organized on a collective basis. On the other hand, a systematic interpretation of the meaning and scope of experience, and yet from two very distinct points of view: the meaning of experience, as studied by the observer (or the psychologist), and experience as known and organized by the subject who constructs his knowledge. The essential feature of classical empiricism is to have given a complete philosophical interpretation of the nature of experience, from this twofold point of view, and of its role in the formation of knowledge, one or two centuries (which is not very long) before the beginnings of a genuine experimental science of perception and intelligence. If many contemporary psychologists continue to support empiricist philosophy, it is above all because of the Anglo-Saxon ideological tradition, just as the psychologists of the USSR are dialecticians, etc. A large number of examples may be quoted to show that as a psychologist one can be a strict experimentalist and interpret the formation of knowledge in an anti-empiricist fashion or independently of empiricist philosophy. The observer's experience can teach him (and has constantly taught me) that knowledge constructed by the subject is not due to experience alone, and that in general it always involves a structuring of which empiricist philosophy has not seen the extent nor grasped the full import.

While Descartes and Leibniz elaborated an epistemology more or less deductively but basing it on already existing sciences, empiricism constructs its own still more or less deductively, by appealing to a science whose scope it only glimpsed and which did not as yet exist. From this there resulted a certain number of lacunae which it is perhaps important to recall briefly in view of the aim of this work and the tendency many readers will have to include its author among the empiricists or positivists.

Firstly, Locke and Hume's arguments against innate ideas are not entirely convincing, for it is still possible that the hereditary structures can manifest themselves not from birth, but by progressive maturation (one then recognizes them from their fixed date of appearance). Such structures can play a part in the formation of concepts and operations, not by including them in advance but by opening up possibilities until then closed (possibilities that will then become actualized by practice).

Secondly, classical empiricism has underestimated the role of logic, whose importance has in part been re-established by contemporary "logical empiricism," although trying to reduce it to a language. Logic, however, proceeds from the general co-ordinations of the subject's actions, which re-establishes the role of the epistemological subject, and thus proportionally diminishes the importance of experience in the ordinary sense (either physical or introspective).

Thirdly, a more precise analysis of the "reading off" of experience and of the mechanisms of learning as a function of experience, teaches us [3] that this "reading off" is always a function of a logico-mathematical framework, which plays a structuring role and not one of simple formulation, that all learning similarly presupposes a logic, and particularly that the learning of logical structures is itself based on logical or preliminary prelogical structures, and this in an endless regress. In short, the experimental study of experience contradicts the interpretations of experience put forward by empiricist philosophy, and this is fundamental if we wish to judge objectively both the contribution of the empiricists in trying to base their philosophy on experience, and the shortcomings of this philosophy.

Fourthly, and finally, when the empiricists decided to study the formation of concepts and thus initiated genetic inquiry, they were satisfied with genetic accounts reconstituted very schematically on an ideal or reflective level. They have over-

---

[3] See Volumes V to X of Etudes d'épistémologie génétique.

looked that the only valid methods in this field are those which systematically make use of historico-critical, sociogenetic, or psychogenetic analyses, and end with comparative studies of historical periods, varied social milieux, and ages of mental development from the child to the adult.

6. If Hume's empiricism, including his associationist interpretations of causality, were pertinent enough to make Kant break away from Leibnizian or Wolffian rationalism, he nevertheless found it inadequate, since it replaced the epistemological subject by knowledge conceived as being a copy of reality. In fact, the most important scientific event of which Kantianism tried to give a general interpretation was anything but a simple copy: the impressive success of the Newtonian doctrine of gravitation and its extension to varied ranges of phenomena was striking evidence of an agreement, even in detail, between logico-mathematical deduction and experience. It was therefore the twofold proof, on the one hand, that the epistemological subject exists and that its constructions form the very stuff of the understanding, and on the other, that experience is structured and even capable of being structured indefinitely, and does not consist in the simple additive collection of recorded facts that satisfied empiricism in its interpretations. It is therefore a question of elaborating a concept of the epistemological subject, satisfying the twofold function of indefinite constructibility and of structuring experience whatever it may be.

Kant has thus originated a fifth kind of epistemological interpretation: that of a-priori construction. But why a priori? We need to recall that prior to Kantianism the choice was, a preformism as yet very static, involving the hypothesis of innate ideas, and the beginnings of a constructivism still very tentative and incomplete, involving the hypothesis of an intellectual attainment as a function of experience. The most natural synthesis consisted therefore in retaining the concept of construction, at least under the form of synthetic judgments, and the idea of innateness, at least under the form of priority as far as experience is concerned. Whence the important idea of synthetic a-priori judgments and the derivative idea that, even in the case of a-posteriori synthetic judgments, intelligence is not limited to receiving impressions like a tabula rasa, but structures reality by means of a-priori forms of sensibility and understanding. It needs to be remembered that the originators of new concepts often give them at first a too rich meaning, the elements of which can be later analyzed out by those who develop their ideas: for example, algebraic operations have been conceived as necessarily commutative before the construction of algebras not having this property, etc. To take account of the agreement of mathematical deduction with experience, in the manner of a pre-established harmony characteristic of epistemological kind IV, but without its somewhat surprising character of static contingency, Kant has therefore elaborated a too rich concept. For it comprises, as it should, universality and necessity (the latter neglected or considered as illusory by empiricism), but also priority in relation to experience: logical priority insofar as it is a necessary condition, as well as priority in part chronological (the a priori can only manifest itself at the moment of experience, and not before, but in all cases not afterward), and above all priority of level, insofar as the subject who experiences already possesses an underlying structure that determines his activities. One can feel very close to the spirit of Kantianism (and I believe I am close to it like many of those who accept the dialectical method) and consider the a priori as dissociable from the notions of chronological priority or of level. The necessity characteristic of the synthesis becomes then a terminus ad quem and ceases to be as in the above case a terminus a quo which still remains too close to the pre-established harmony. More precisely, the construction characteristic of the epistemological subject, however rich it is in the Kantian perspective, is still too poor, since it is completely given at the start. On the other hand, a dialectical construction, as seen in the history of science and in the experimental facts brought to light by studies on mental development, seems to show the living reality. It enables us to attribute to the epistemological subject a much richer constructivity, although ending with the same characteristics of rational necessity and the structuring of experience, as those which Kant called for to guarantee his concept of the *a priori*.

7. The important philosophical systems whose connections with science we have just noted have been constructed by their originators in the context of a science either already constituted (before or by them), or glimpsed by them before it had been constituted (biology for Aristotle, who also founded logic, and psychology for classical empiricism). To the latter belongs Hegel's dialectic (sixth kind of epistemology), which arose under the influence of historical and sociological thought, and which exhibits its novelty in relation to the essentially conceptual use that Kant already made of the dialectic. Hegel cannot be made the founder of sociology any more than the empiricists can be made the founders of psychology, but it seems clear that a concern for sociological knowledge has played with him the same role as the concern for psychological knowledge among the empiricists. If the dialectic remained an integral part of the post-Kantian idealism, its fundamental concept of a concrete universal has, as is well known, played its part in the constitution of the Marxian dialectic. On the other hand, if Hegel's system is no exception to the rule according to which the most important doctrines in the history of philosophy have arisen from a reflection on the possibility of a science already established or simply anticipated, the need for speculation, reinforced and not checked by the Kantian critique of purely theoretical reason which found its support in the idealist interpretation of the transcendental self, did not remain alien to Hegel. While opening the way to the concrete universal in the domain of mind, he has in that of nature given one of the best examples of speculative reason of a parascientific tendency, that is to say, one pursuing the ideal of a form of knowledge properly so called which would duplicate science in its own domain. The *Naturphilosophie* thus remains an example giving cause for thought, for it is one thing to take up a reflective point of view in the case of a science which does not yet exist, as did the empiricists in their

approach to psychology, and quite another to duplicate an already existing science. This raises the question of the duality of possible knowledge about the same subject matter and the legitimacy of statements accepted as knowledge by some and not by others. We shall come across this problem again in the case of contemporary philosophical psychology, that is to say, not that psychology which gave rise to scientific psychology, but that which claims to duplicate or even to replace it.

8. We shall not refer here to Bergson and Husserl, with whom we will deal in Chapters Three and Four, for the epistemology of the first has not been followed up and that of the second has become an integral part of a´ general system which states in a most direct way the problem of the duality of knowledge (spatio-temporal, or "of the world," and "eidetic"), which will call for a more detailed examination in Chapter Three. Let us simply note for the moment that this epistemology, very interesting in itself because it goes back to a position intermediate between kinds I and II, but with the addition of a transcendental self, originates like the others from the progress of a particular science. Husserl had begun in his *Philosophie der Arithmetik* by making use of psychology in the form of a reference to a certain number of basic mental operations (one of which is colligation). But after having been criticized by logicians and under Frege's influence, he has immersed himself in the latter's work and thus discovered the need to get away from the spatio-temporal. From this arises the famous phenomenological "reduction," "bracketing," and the whole of the anti-psychologism that became current in the logistic domain.

(D) These few schematic remarks (and I apologize for this rather loosely knit account, but it perhaps suffices for the moment) show the existence of two important dominating trends in the history of philosophy, one relatively constant and the other variable. The former is the set of problems that are concerned with the meaning of human life in relation to the whole of reality: that which we refer to by the phrase "problems of the coordination of values." If one can speak about the relative constant it is certainly not the case that every metaphysic has adopted the same solutions to these problems, since the latter are, on the contrary, those about which agreement is impossible because of the irreducibility of the value judgments distinguishing different tendencies, such as, for example, mentalism and materialism. But there is a relative constancy in the sense that the important metaphysical positions are relatively few and have remained the same throughout history, without one seeing, despite Leibniz's efforts or the eclecticisms of all intellectual levels, how they could be reconciled.

The dominating variable tendency, considered in the preceding remarks (C), is the problem of knowledge, for in order to include human life and theological questions within the whole of reality, we need a cognitive position and not merely a praxological one. There is thus an initial tendency for the synthesis of knowledge, which is quickly centered on what has become the essential question, that of the very nature and scope of knowledge. It is with respect to this dominant epistemology that one can speak of variations in the sense of innumerable lines of progress, yet marked by the most varied directional changes. Such progress, which generally shows itself as a passage from realism to constructivism, has formed an integral part of the history of science. It has been due either to a reflection on an existing science accepted as such, or to the discovery of lacunae and to the anticipation of sciences still to be constituted (as biology for Aristotle, in contrast to logic, which he had founded, psychology for empiricism and sociology for the dialectic). For the great philosophical innovators of the past there was therefore no opposition between science and philosophy, either they have also been innovators in the field of science itself (and we have seen under B how, in those thinkers who were both scientists and philosophers, these two aspects of their work influenced each other in manifold ways: from whence the positions characteristic of C5 and 7), or they have accepted an already existing science.

The elaboration of systems having for their goal the attainment of philosophical knowledge *sui generis* and distinct from scientific knowledge, is therefore only a relatively recent phenomenon, and we shall need to examine the historical reasons for this. Spinoza's impressive work, which is concerned entirely with the coordination of values, has no such pretension, and his *Ethics* proceeds *more geometrico* without having to start with an opposition between *Geisteswissenschaften* and natural science. More recently, although Höffding's work has been largely taken up with a pure immanentism, his very different approach to the religious problem has not prevented him from constructing a profound philosophy of religion without having to duplicate on the cognitive level his scientific habits by developing a specific mode of philosophical knowledge. Apart from a few exceptions like Höffding, Cassirer, Brunschvicg, etc., there has hardly been a philosophy of mind since the nineteenth century which has not tried to base itself not only on special methods, but on a mode of knowledge conceived as peculiar to philosophy, and as alien to all scientific knowledge.

On the other hand, it is only at a relatively recent date (and the two phenomena are clearly connected, but resulting from a complex interaction and not a one-way causality) that some scientists lacking a philosophical training have engaged in philosophical speculation without knowing it. Instead of thinking about the epistemological conditions of their subject (or of scientific systems in general), they have believed they could derive directly from it a dogmatic materialism or some other philosophy.

These different signs of a tragic divorce of the different forms of knowledge, and in many respects of the human mind itself, are clear evidence of the increasing importance since the nineteenth century of a similar general phenomenon. With the very rapid increase in and disproportionate specialization of branches of knowledge, one and the same scholar can no longer be in touch with them all, but still (and one is less aware of this) neither can he obtain for himself an adequate idea of the specialized epistemologies based on them. The "theory of knowledge" only has a general value and serious interest for us if it takes account of all the special forms of epistemology as a function of the differentiation of knowledge itself. The twofold phenomenon of parascientific philosophies and of metaphysical scientists thus depends (without prejudging particular factors to which we will return in Chapter Three) on this general factor of the increasing difficulty of the epistemological material. But this lack of adequate knowledge of other epistemologies is always to be seen more clearly in others than in ourselves. We can each see that if Haeckel or Le Dantec had thought about the epistemology of mathematics, their materialism might have been less naïve, but we see much less clearly that if Husserl had been sufficiently aware of the possibilities of genetic psychology he would have had no need of "eidetic" knowledge in order to resolve the problem of how we arrive at nontemporal structures. Further, this forced introversion of each thinker or school is again increased among philosophers by the absence of the habit of interdisciplinary work, which is becoming widespread among scientists and is their chief safeguard against scientific and above all epistemological compartmentalization. It is hard to believe that Daval and Guillebaud's excellent little book on *Le raisonnement mathématique*, resulting from the collaboration of a philosopher and the most subtle of mathematicians interested in the human sciences, has not been followed up, as if philosophical reflection implied fixation on the self.

(E) To anyone concerned with seeing that knowledge is soundly based rather than with philosophical or scientific labels, and who hopes to remedy the present confusion by bringing about a much closer agreement between thinkers, two complementary ways of approach seem open. On the one hand, one can return to the origins so as to rediscover the tendencies that were in process of development before the tragic divorce of science and philosophical reflection, and on the other, there is the possibility of an organized or organic differentiation of problems such that their specialized delimitation requires synthesis, in opposition to the general global or syncretic conceptions which have for their aim the totality of things, and end in fact at a multiplication of schools no longer speaking the same language. This delimitation of problems seems to coincide precisely with those tendencies discernible among the great thinkers of the past, at periods where professional philosophy was not open to anyone and was bound up with the careers of thinkers who had begun by learning how to solve particular problems.

The classical problems of philosophy can be grouped under five main heads: 1) the search for the absolute, or metaphysics; 2) the normative noncognitive disciplines like ethics and aesthetics; 3) logic, or the theory of formal norms of knowledge; 4) psychology and sociology; 5) epistemology, or the general theory of knowledge. Let us therefore try to see under what conditions it would be possible in these different fields to arrive at, not a *consensus* or a common opinion, which always runs the risk of only resulting from suggestion, authority, etc., but a progress in cooperation between thinkers initially in disagreement. We have here only an external sign of knowledge, but the analysis of the procedures used to arrive at such an agreement can lead to more intrinsic information, when it is a question of methods of argumentation so excellently analyzed by C. Perelman, or of intersubjective methods of testing or verification.

1. As a subject metaphysics, together with psychology and scientific sociology, has the doubtful privilege that some people believe in it and others do not. A society of metaphysicians could come to agree on some extremely general principles, such as the existence of a boundary, between metaphysical problems and others, although they will fail to agree as to where the boundary is to be drawn and on its fixed or variable character. But the analogy ends here. When two psychologists disagree about a particular problem, which, of course, often happens, they can only, if personality factors do not enter to cause misunderstanding, be activated by an honest disagreement, since it will lead them to learn something about the facts and their interpretation. When two metaphysicians disagree, however honest and well-intentioned they may be, this disagreement depends, if there is no

misunderstanding, on questions of conviction and not of verification or of logic. One can lessen the disagreement by clever argument, by an appeal to common values: it cannot be reduced by a factual verification or a formal demonstration. If there existed for such metaphysical questions tests that were able to convince everyone, we would then speak of truth, pure and simple, and no longer of metaphysics. Descartes regarded the proposition *Je pense donc je suis* as incontrovertible, and my teacher Reymond saw in the *Cogito* the verification of a metaphysical hypothesis. But verification of what? If it is a question of clarifying the metaphysical meaning of "thinking" and "existing," the verifications become vague. If, on the other hand, it is a question of asserting that all knowledge is dependent on the existence of a subject: this is then the important discovery of the epistemological subject, but we are now concerned with epistemology and no longer with metaphysics.

It would be unwise to try to give advice to metaphysicians, but let us assume that as a former president of the International Union of Scientific Psychology [4] or as a member of the International Institute of Philosophy (to which I proudly belong) I am asked together with others to cooperate in a project among metaphysicians of all schools, selected so as to be as widely representative and complete as possible. I would then suggest the following research program:

(a) Each individual should state in the most explicit form possible (in terms of a set of hypotheses or axioms) three to ten of the most important of his metaphysical theses.

(b) For each thesis he should state, as honestly as he can, whether he thinks it to be demonstrable, given intuitively, or due to intimate convictions going beyond the field of knowledge.

(c) In the case of such convictions to state their moral, social, and religious nature, etc.

---

[4] The latter has made a habit of collaboration, and is at the moment proceeding with projects of comparative psychology in different countries and cultural milieux.

(d) In the case of intuition to specify the level: immediate, transcendental, etc.

(e) In the case where a thesis seems to be demonstrable to give this demonstration in a rough form and to distinguish explicitly: 1) reference to facts; 2) reference to rational norms, indicating their nature; 3) the procedure of logical deduction.

(f) These sets of answers are then to be seen by each member of the group and each is to indicate for the preceding points of the others' theses his agreement or disagreement in terms of a qualitative scale graduated as follows: valid, more or less probable (or plausible), undecidable, and unacceptable.

The sets of answers thus evaluated would not, of course, lead to a value judgment on the theses themselves, but to useful information as to the existing state of agreement and disagreement about them, and particularly about the degrees of truth given by the subjects to their own metaphysical judgments or to those of others. Such a comparison would then be the starting point for wider comparative studies, which would lead on the one hand to the further extension of C. Perelman's researches on argumentation (it would specifically concern metaphysical argument), and on the other hand, to an epistemological analysis. The latter would no doubt lead us to distinguish degrees of knowledge (just as many logical systems place between truth and falsity a series of values of probability and decidability), and especially those kinds of knowledge that are a function of our noncognitive values (ethical, religious, etc.), but which are held as certain, or probable, etc. It would then become possible without upsetting anyone's susceptibilities, to distinguish in addition to strict knowledge, that which one would call "wisdom" (σοφία), i.e. all the kinds of plausible knowledge grouped as a function of a general coordination of values.

Moreover, such an epistemological and comparative analysis could only be of help to sociological studies, such as those of L. Goldmann on Kant or on Jansenism, showing the relationship between a philosophy or a theology and the social structures they partly reflect. From such a point of view, the mode of thought which is characteristic of a form of wisdom appears to come close to symbolic thought, but the mythical and image content of the latter is replaced by concepts which, although of different degrees of abstraction, include individual or social values not contained in their cognitive definition.

2. The position of ethics as a branch of philosophy may vary according to the moral philosopher, from a definite subordination to metaphysics, to an independence based on the study of "moral experience" in Frederic Rauh's sense. The latter position is an extremely fruitful one and has this advantage, for anyone who believes that a progressive intersubjective agreement is the sole corrective which can serve as a check upon individual thought, it gives an analytical tool for all types of morality including metaphysical ones, while the converse is not true.

But the great difference between the two points of view is that Rauh's method returns to the study of the morality of the subject: norms forming an integral part of an autonomous system, or of a revelation, etc. The situation seems therefore comparable with that of logic, where one can also distinguish (and where this has also to be done with care) the subject's logic and that of the logician or logic pure and simple. Except that in the case of logic, the subject's norms are inconsistent and "natural logic" is very poor. The question whether the logician's logic is to start off with thought derived from the subject's mental operations, while at the same time giving rise by means of the axiomatic method to a rich and autonomous constructive development, concerns psychology and epistemology but is of no interest to logic. For the latter once set up axiomatically becomes completely independent of mental facts (except in explaining its boundaries, such as the "limits of formalization"). In the case of ethics, on the contrary, the subject's morality forms the supreme criterion, and the great historical ethical systems originate from the "moral experience" of exceptional personalities, like Christ or Buddha.

Is it necessary to conclude from this that the work of every moral philosopher endeavoring to prescribe norms is useless unless he does this either by communicating or trying to convince others of his own personal experience? And that his inferiority in relation to the logician (who prescribes from the sole fact that he demonstrates without being concerned to give advice) is final and irremediable? We do not think so, we have here a very extensive field of inquiry that has hardly yet been opened up. Rauh's "moral experience" provides us with a table of the subject's norms, and of variable norms, for there exists a large number of individual and group moralities. There is therefore no reason why we should not formalize these norms, in terms of a logic of values, as we can formalize the particular structures of natural thought, so as to compare them with the structures of logic (of logicians). In the case of ethics, where what is really of interest is the subject's morality, and not that of the moral philosopher, a comparison between the different formalized moralities of the subject could give valuable information about what these structures have in common and the passage from one to the other. Further, and this is of direct interest to general problems, even an elementary formalization enables one to draw a boundary between the field of interpersonal exchanges, spontaneous and nonnormative, that of qualitative values (sympathies, esteem, prestige, etc.), and exchanges involving a necessary conservation of values (normative reciprocity, etc.). The latter correspond to what one usually calls moral relations or exchanges.[5]

Such formalizations will deal, of course, with questions of structure, and they will be related to decision problems that are fundamental in the subject's morality. R. B. Braithwaite, Emeritus Professor of Moral Philosophy at the University of Cambridge, has in this connection written an extremely suggestive little book on *Ethics and the Theory of Games*. This mathematical theory due to the economist Morgenstern and the mathematician Von Neumann, is also called decision theory and

[5] I have tried to show this in an *Essai sur la théorie des valeurs qualitatives en sociologie statique*, reproduced in *Etudes sociologiques*, Geneva (Droz), 1965.

provides models, which are at once extremely concrete and extremely general, of choice and decision. What Braithwaite has done is to show their relation to moral problems.

2(a). Moral philosophy has many connections with that of law. In a general fashion one can distinguish in the exchanges of values between human beings four important categories. There are at first the spontaneous nonnormative exchanges, which comprise two categories: that of social qualitative values, which we have just considered, and that of quantified values, which is a factor in economic exchanges. With regard to normative exchanges, they also include two categories: moral exchanges and juridical ones, one of their differences being that the latter is codified at all levels, from the interindividual contract to state codification.

Let us simply note here that the philosophies of law can similarly be arranged according to different levels, starting from the extreme of metaphysical dependence to complete independence. In the case of the metaphysics of law, some systems of which are bound up with a religious position, it is interesting to note that the concept of "natural law," constructed initially as a reaction against the divine right of kings, etc., has, on the contrary, become today plainly metaphysical by reaction now to positive law, and which would in some cases merit rather the name of supernatural law. With regard to autonomous theories of law, we find as in ethics the danger of a psychologism or a sociologism that would make their normative characteristics vanish. On the other hand, in order to retain the latter in their essential importance, as is the case in logic and ethics, we find in the admirable normative system constructed by Kelsen a solution that not only meets with increased favor among jurists, but also gives the epistemologist the exceptional opportunity of possible formalization and of relating it to ethical and logical structures.

2(b). We know that aesthetics also encounters similar problems and that alongside philosophical aesthetics there has developed a scientific aesthetics, which endeavors to analyze the objective and subjective conditions entering into aesthetic judgments of various kinds.

3. Logic is the striking example of a branch of philosophy that has become almost from the start independent of metaphysics, developed without conflict as an independent discipline (with increasing help from sciences alien to philosophy, like mathematics), and which nevertheless, or rather because of its independent development, has helped and will increasingly be of help to all branches of philosophy.

Peripatetic logic, which together with Aristotelian philosophy, originated in an intellectual climate as metaphysical as it was biological, was little influenced by metaphysics, since the syllogistic had the rare distinction of being found valid from the start. However, the Aristotelian theory of substance and attributes has had a limiting effect on this rapid development, and has stood in the way of a conscious realization of the logic of relations to the exclusive advantage of that of classes and syllogistic inclusions.

Subsequently, and in spite of some local progress (Stoic logic, Buridan's discovery of the disjunction, Leibniz's intuitions, etc.), logic has remained somewhat static until the renaissance due to the work of Hamilton, Jevons, Boole, de Morgan, etc., *i.e.* until its mathematization and the discovery of Boolean algebra based upon the calculus of propositions. From this time onward one could certainly speak of an opposition between philosophical logic faithful to the scholastic tradition and scientific or mathematical logic, but this was only a manner of speaking and did not hide any real conflict, like that existing today between scientific psychology and philosophical psychology. On the one hand, philosophy teachers cannot claim that the new logic is false: they simply neglect it, in which they are followed by the textbooks with their usual delay, and cannot thus prevent it from having an independence in some way forced upon them. On the other hand, logicians do not claim that the syllogistic is false (apart from one or two apparent errors due simply to a defect in clarity of exposition), they can only point out its inadequate formalization and insufficient generality.

However, in spite of or because of this independence, a necessary condition for its progress since the nineteenth century, logic has been of great value to philosophy, since it provided it with the example of a consistent normative discipline, as well as giving its technical aid to every kind of formalization. The metaphysicians concerned with absolute norms took logic as a model without at all impeding its progress, since these norms do not enter into the technical work of axiomatization. The antipsychologism of Husserl, etc., took its model from logic without impeding it either, since its methods remain alien in principle to any appeal to mental facts, etc.

Finally, logic forms a necessary framework of reference for epistemology to which the latter can refer as a paradigm as far as formal and deductive consistency is concerned, in opposition to questions of fact relative to the subject's activities.

4. Psychology, a factual science, has only achieved its independence at a much later date than logic, a deductive science, for the same reasons that experimental physics only developed centuries after mathematics. The first of these is that if the norms, the antecedents and consequents, of an argument, implications, etc., can be directly grasped by the mind that can analyze them in manipulating them, an experimental fact necessitates, on the contrary, the isolation of factors that cannot be obtained deductively and presupposes a controlled experiment, in opposition to the brute facts of immediate experience, which are invariably misleading. The second reason is that a scientific fact always involves an interpretation. This is firstly because it is an answer to a preliminary question, and to ask a question presupposes an intellectual elaboration, then because the "reading off" and the giving of form to it implies a structuring, which is bound up with a system of hypotheses that has led to the question and is to a greater or lesser extent subject to revision as a function of the answers. Contrary to commonsense opinion, it is hence much more difficult to verify facts and to analyze

them than to reflect or perform deductions. This is why the experimental sciences originate long after the deductive disciplines, the latter forming both the framework and the necessary conditions of the former, but not the sufficient.

Consequently, psychology for long consisted in scattered observations and analyses carried out by philosophers during their studies, which was undoubtedly one of the sources of scientific psychology. Together with a deceptive terminology and speculations about the soul, one finds in the great philosophers a large number of fruitful ideas that have since then given rise to systematic investigations. But in spite of the fundamental remarks of Kant on the self as a unity of apperception excluding all substantialism, pre-scientific psychology has often been used for idealistic speculations. Because of this, when scientific psychology became an independent discipline it for long distrusted the direct study of the higher intellectual functions, and at first concerned itself with problems of sensation, perception, association, etc., in a psycho-physiological context. This situation has produced an understandable conflict, and its persistence leads to increasing absurdities among those thinkers who see interesting problems, but treat them from a bird's-eye view without respecting the rules of verification, and those who bring them under an experimental discipline but excessively restrict their field. From this has arisen the idea, inconceivable in other fields, of a philosophical psychology able to duplicate scientific psychology, finding an additional motivation in the very legitimate philosophical need for the coordination of values (as if a "philosophical anthropology" could be satisfied with knowledge on the cheap).

This problem is much too important for us to limit ourselves to only a few remarks about it: the whole of Chapter Four will be concerned with its examination.

5. There remains the theory of knowledge, which has been the great contribution of philosophical thought from Plato down to almost all contemporary thinkers. The question we shall examine here is whether by the nature of its problems it

has necessarily to remain linked with metaphysics or whether it exhibits, either in principle or in fact (nonexclusive disjunction), tendencies toward independence, as has been the case with logic and psychology.

In principle, it seems clear that epistemology is supreme, for in wishing to construct a metaphysics we have to answer the preliminary questions whether metaphysical knowledge is possible and under what conditions. We have had, however, to wait for Kant for these questions to be stated in all their generality, and he has answered the first in the negative as far as pure theoretical reason is concerned, and he has substituted for dogmatic metaphysics what one can call a "wisdom" based on pure practical reason. This wisdom has, moreover, been so ephemeral that the post-Kantians have had nothing more pressing to do than to transform the critical apparatus into an absolute self, etc.

Epistemology has, in fact, shown all the usual signs of a tendency toward independence: delimitation of problems, constitution of internal methods of verification, and contributions from already constituted sciences.

The delimitation of problems has begun with Descartes, Leibniz, and Kant; the latter gave under a static form an exhaustive and definitive table of a-priori forms of sensibility and a-priori schemes of the understanding. From this has resulted a number of special problems that have increasingly become more delimited in character. For example, the highly debatable solution that Kant gives of the problem of number in basing it on time and not merely on the categories of quantity of the understanding, has been taken up by Brouwer, who has turned it into a method opposed to the logical reductionism of Frege, Whitehead, and Russell (an example, moreover, of the passage from a general epistemological problem to an increasingly specialized mathematical and logical epistemology). Further, the Kantian interpretation of space as an a-priori form of sensibility has led to two important classes of investigations. One has been followed by the first experimental psychologists, who were not so ignorant of the main philosophical problems as is sometimes believed. Since it is a question of "sensibility," verification was possible and important psycho-physiologists like Müller and Hering have explicitly maintained the Kantian thesis, under the name of "nativism," against the "empiricism" of Helmholtz (who, moreover, introduced unconscious inferences even in perception). The problem has continued, nevertheless, to be studied on the experimental field and spatial constructivism, which seems to imply it is much closer to Kantianism given a dynamic interpretation than a pure empiricism. On the other hand, the discovery of non-Euclidean geometries has contradicted the letter but not the spirit of a priorism (as is well known, Poincaré, despite his conventionalism, made the concept of a "group" an a-priori structure) and has given rise to a completely specialized geometrical epistemology.

This specialization of problems, which has steadily increased (when one thinks, for example, of the work of E. Meyerson, which is entirely given up to epistemology), has naturally led to an increasing accuracy of methods concerned with substituting verification for simple reflection. In the field of deductive demonstration, progress has been very great, although much less but still considerable in the field of facts. And in both cases progress has exhibited itself, among other ways, in the increasingly important contributions coming from science itself, and no longer only from the professional philosopher.

In the field of deductive analysis, the independent development of logic has produced two large groups of studies, which have become fundamental for mathematical epistemology and whose increasing technical nature has transformed the latter into a branch of mathematics itself, concerned with the theory of its foundations (to such an extent that today almost every International Congress of Mathematics has a whole section devoted to this new field). The first of these groups of studies has been concerned with the problem of the possible reduction of mathematics to logic. This possibility, brilliantly stated in Whitehead and Russell's *Principia Mathematica* but questioned by others, has been studied under all its aspects, while the work of a second group of investigators, particularly Hilbert, Ackermann, and Bernays, has tried to demonstrate the noncontradictory character of fundamental parts of mathematics like arithmetic. These diverse investigations ended about 1930 in Gödel's discovery of theorems, which have marked a decisive turning point in mathematical epistemology, and whose general import is the impossibility of demonstrating the noncontradiction of a theory by its own methods or by weaker methods. From this results the important idea of a constructivism such that, in order to guarantee the consistency of the initial theories it is necessary to include them in higher-order theories, which themselves are similarly dependent on other theories, etc. One sees the epistemological importance of such a conception, which contradicts both Platonism and positivist reductionism in favor of a constructivism glimpsed by many philosophers, but henceforth supported by a richer and more precise internal epistemology.

In the field of facts, an important trend has been discernible among French-speaking epistemologists, while Anglo-Saxon empiricism has raised other problems. After the distinguished studies of Cournot—whose true value has for so long been neglected—which dealt with the analysis of scientific thought in a somewhat synchronic perspective, a certain number of thinkers like G. Milhaud, L. Brunschvicg, P. Boutroux, and A. Reymond, have realized that the epistemological significance of a scientific theory only fully shows itself when seen in its historical perspective. This is so because it answers the questions raised by earlier doctrines and prepares the way for its successors by a network of relationships that continue or contradict it. In other words, as scientific thought is continually developing, the problem of what knowledge is can only be resolved under the most limited forms, which tend to analyze the way in which knowledge grows or develops in the context of actual construction. From this results the historico-critical method, one of the most important methods of scientific epistemology.

But, in addition, a large number of writers have propounded problems about facts in the most diverse fields. In that of mathematical epistemology, F. Enriques looked for the explanation of different structures in the operations of thought and for the different geometries in the different perceptual ranges, and H. Poincaré derived the group of displacements from sensori-motor organization. In the physical field, while physicists discuss their own epistemological problems resulting from the question of the relations between the observer, reality, and the observable, the "logical empiricists," who continue the tradition of classical empiricism, elaborate a synthetic theory of judgment based upon perceptual verification, in opposition to analytic judgments based upon a logico-mathematical language, etc.

We therefore had the idea of studying the problem of the development and growth of knowledge going back to its psychogenetic formation, and this for two reasons. On the one hand, it is a natural extension of the historico-critical method. P. Boutroux, for example, retraces the history of mathematics, showing how we have passed from the "contemplative" period of the Greeks to one of "synthesis," *i.e.* of operational combination, then to a period where the "intrinsic objectivity" of these operational structures is discovered. The first problem is to see whether these structures exhibit natural origins corresponding to the general structures of intelligence, or whether they arise from purely technical constructions. Such a problem can only be dealt with on the psychogenetic field; adult introspection gives no information on this matter. On the other hand, since the empiricists and their modern followers have brought in, rightly or wrongly, psychological mechanisms in order to explain at least some aspects of knowledge—perceptual experience for physical knowledge, language for logico-mathematical structures, etc.—it is now time to verify the value of such explanations in these fields of inquiry, and here again only psychogenetic studies are illuminating.

In this way genetic epistemology originated an essentially interdisciplinary field of research that endeavors to study the meaning of forms of knowledge, of operational structures or of concepts, by referring on the one hand to their history and to their present functioning in some determinate science (this information being given by specialists in that science and in its epistemology); on the other, to their logical aspect (by reference to logicians), and finally to their psychogenetic formation or their relations with mental structures (this aspect giving rise to the investigations of professional psychologists interested also in epistemology). Epistemology thus conceived is no longer a matter of simple reflection, but in endeavoring to study knowledge in its growth (for this formation is itself a mechanism of growth, without an absolute beginning) and assuming that such growth always simultaneously gives rise to questions of fact and norms, it tries to combine the only adequate methods for deciding such questions. These are, on the one hand, that of logic, which no one would question in its specialized form, and, on the other, that of the history of ideas and the psychology of their development, the latter having been constantly introduced implicitly or explicitly, but always under its experimental and specialized form in questions of intelligence properly so called.

Although the above outline is extremely schematic it suffices to show that epistemology starting from philosophical reflection has through its own technical progress tended to become independent of metaphysics. This independence has been achieved in contrast to psychology without an overt declaration of aims, and is more comparable with that which has marked the evolution of logic. Scientific epistemology is, however, much less advanced because its major studies have only been undertaken fairly recently by investigators concerned with other studies without their being able to concentrate exclusively on epistemological analysis. This is especially the case because to carry out an effective epistemological investigation almost necessarily presupposes interdisciplinary collaboration.

The general conclusion to be drawn from 1 to 5 above is that, leaving on one side metaphysics, all philosophical inquiries deal with problems capable of being delimited, and which tend to become differentiated under forms approximating ever more closely to those of scientific inquiry. This is because the differences between science and philosophy are not due to the nature of the problems, but to their delimitation and to the increasing technical nature of their methods of verification. But this is not the view of most philosophers. In Chapters Three and Four we will therefore try to examine other positions concerning these central problems of method.

The False Ideal
of a Suprascientific
Knowledge

Chapter Three

WE HAVE SEEN in the last chapter that science and philosophy were once not in conflict and noted some of the methods that have been used, or are still being evolved, to re-establish harmony between them by a delimitation or specialization of problems. We have now to consider the much more serious situation, which is the origin of real conflict and which arose during the nineteenth century, when some philosophers believed they possessed a *sui generis* mode of knowledge superior to that of science. It is with respect to this parascientific "knowledge," claimed to be suprascientific, that we need to take up a definite position.

(A) Let us again consider an example from the field of finality [see Chapter Two under (A)]. I know some very intelligent philosophers, not at all dogmatic, who believe that "science" cannot introduce the concept of finality in the analysis and explanation of vital processes, but that "philosophy" equally cannot arrive at an adequate concept of organic life without introducing finality. It is not a question here of moral or other values, but rather of a concept peculiar to philosophical biology as opposed to biology. Indeed, one such philosopher concluded, drawing inspiration from Merleau-Ponty, that science can "never" give an adequate explanation of the concept of the "whole structure" of the organism.

Without for the moment referring to phenomenology, and remaining on the ground of simple common sense, what do such statements, relatively widespread today, mean? They would have astonished a Cartesian or a Leibnizian, since they deny or "accept" finality but in the scientific and philosophical fields at one and the same time. The problem here is not that of finality, but rather the duality of modes of knowledge for the subject. Undoubtedly, the concept of finality is obscure: attraction at a distance and infinite velocity, which Newtonian gravitation appeared to prescribe, were obscurer still, but it seemed to constitute either a fact or an almost unavoidable interpretation of fact (and we cannot escape this by asserting it to be philosophically true and scientifically false or vice versa). The question is: How can we assert that a concept is both unacceptable and acceptable, or even necessary, and for the same things, but depending on whether they are considered scientifically or philosophically? It is plain that two modes of knowledge are postulated, one of which is higher than the other, because it attains the essential, while the other is "lower," as it is either merely verbal or incomplete knowledge, limited by certain boundaries (spatio-temporal, etc.) or by certain principles (positivist, etc.). But if there exists a superior kind of knowledge, which comprises everything including the inferior kind, and an inferior knowledge inevitably limited, why not explain this? This is just what is happening, and there are many philosophically inclined biologists who are finalists. But a serious problem then arises: why has this not led to any progress?

The seriousness of this problem is due to the fact that the word "truth" is taken in two different senses. It is intellectually intolerable to admit that there exist two kinds of truth, for logic requires their coordination. To say that for perception the sun moves around a visible region of the earth and that for reason the earth moves around the sun, these are, if one wishes to put it in this way, two truths, but relative to levels of phenomena that are easy to coordinate. To assert, on the contrary, that the structure of the organism can only be grasped by philosophical

G

intuition and implies among other things "finality," and that the honest biologist working day after day in his laboratory (and with methods that yield results) cannot understand this, since he is limited by an heuristic and conceptual blindness so that these intuitions are unavailable to him, this is no longer to refer to different but coordinatable levels. It is coldly to cut human thought into two heterogeneous parts, and to alter the very meaning of the word "truth" so as to give it two incompatible meanings.

The ordinary meaning of the word "truth" refers to that which is verifiable by everyone. The method of verification does not much matter provided it is open to all, and guarantees for the subject that it is not centered on his self or on the authority of a master, but that the position he puts forward can be verified by anyone who questions it. If the finality of the organism was "true" in this sense, even if it was not verifiable by means of the microscope, and that in order to attain it it was necessary to make an effort of deduction and abstraction as difficult as one might wish, and for which rules could be given, this would be a truth nonetheless. It would be a scientific truth, understood by an élite only, but open to anyone willing to perform the necessary labor. To say, on the contrary, that finality is forced on "philosophy" is deliberately to overlook that there are a large number of philosophies other than one's own, and that neither Descartes nor Spinoza nor the modern dialectic had the advantage of these intuitions. The "truth" condition, in the second sense of the term, is therefore no longer verification resulting from either a deduction or a method open to all, but arrived at by means of persuasion or conversion, *i.e.* by the acceptance of a system. Of course, algebra is a system, biology is also one, etc.: then why not Bergsonism or phenomenology? Simply because some of us have scruples in believing before being certain, or in calling something true that still involves an element of belief, even considered as self-evident, when it concerns "self-evidences" that are peculiar to others or, by analogy, to oneself.

(B) But perhaps these are only affective reactions, and in a world where subjective "existence" has become the source of truth, it is possible that systems, which at the very least exist, could be tomorrow's truth. Let us therefore try to understand the factors that have given rise to the tendency to accept a mode of knowledge peculiar to philosophy and superior to scientific knowledge. We will then try to consider the reasons, given among others, by phenomenology, which is much the most distinguished of the systems based on such a belief.

1. The first observable factor is undoubtedly the search for the absolute. As long as there was no conflict between science and philosophy, metaphysics could appear as the supreme synthesis, comprising all knowledge and without requiring a special mode of knowledge in order to transcend the particular disciplines. Starting from the decisive turning point marked by the Kantian critique, which denied to theoretical reason the right to go beyond the bounds of structuring reality, the heroism of such a position has not been sufficient to overcome the need for the absolute. His followers have seen in the a-priori structures no longer an epistemological table of the conditions of knowledge, in accordance with its Kantian stringency, but the expression of a power peculiar to philosophical thought, which, in determining the preliminary methods necessary for science, places itself above it. Together with the need for the absolute there resulted a suprascientific position, no longer by synthesis but by a delimitation of levels.

It is unnecessary to recall the many expressions of this same tendency, which consists under all its forms in restricting scientific knowledge within certain limits constitutive of "phenomena" and to search for the foundations of such a limited mode of knowledge in order to attain a mode of a higher level. As against this it is important to note that such a process, perfectly legitimate in itself, can give rise to procedures, either purely speculative, or systematic and verified. Under this last form, the fundamental process of the differentiation of levels is not alien to the sciences themselves and it is a fundamental error to assume that their data are to be found on one and the same level. Considering only physics, for example, "phenomena" occur on different levels, not because they are there completely organized and that, according to our use of the microscope or telescope, they appear different, but because according to the profound remark of C. Eugène Guye, it is the level that creates the phenomena. In other words, physics concerns itself with a series of structures each of which can be considered as knowledge of a higher level in relation to the preceding ones. On the other hand, from the establishment of laws to their causal or deductive explanation, characteristic of "theoretical physics," and from the latter to that pure and autonomous deductive system constituted by "mathematical physics" (in respect of which A. Lichnerovicz has shown in his studies and S. Bachelard in an excellent historico-critical analysis how much it differs from theoretical physics), there is a new change of planes or of level, of such a kind that the initial phenomena eventually become integrated within a conceptual universe including all possibilities and no longer only reality. Finally, when a science like mathematics includes within its domain its own epistemology under the form of a systematic and scientific analysis of its foundations, it is clear that one and the same discipline thus multiplies internally its own levels of construction and reflection.

By wishing to restrict science within certain boundaries in order to facilitate the belief in the possibility of a specific and superior mode of knowledge, the parascientific philosophies are therefore always in danger of seeing these boundaries constantly change, and their own field of inquiry encroached upon by otherwise sounder methods.

2. On the other hand, there is a second general reason that explains the parascientific tendencies and which still arises from the need for speculation, but this time among scientists themselves. Such a need is due, in fact, to human nature and philosophers have the advantage, when they succumb to it, that they also possess a historical training, which enables them to make a general survey of existing theories before finding new ones.

When some nineteenth-century scientists, especially biologists without a mathematical, logical, or psychological training, have wanted to extend their growing knowledge into a metaphysics, they have accepted a dogmatic materialism that has influenced the ordinary man more (without speaking of social factors) as it appeared to derive simply from science itself. The surprising thing is that philosophers have been victims of the same illusion, so that as a reaction against materialism they have proceeded to criticize science.

A critique of scientific knowledge is termed an epistemology, and every epistemological study is to be welcomed whatever be its purpose. Thus the famous work of E. Boutroux on *La contingence des lois de la nature* is of great interest as a critique of the ideal of absolute deduction and as a refutation of reductionism. From this point of view the subsequent advance of science has shown the correctness of his position. It increasingly appears that wherever one has arrived at a reduction of the higher to the lower, or the more complex to the more simple, this reduction becomes reciprocal, *i.e.* the lower is enriched by certain characteristics of the higher and the "more simple" as such becomes more complex. Thus in reducing gravitation to spatial-curvature, which seemed to be a reduction of the physical to the geometrical, Einstein has been led to relate this curvature to mass in such a way that the reduction is reciprocal. As C. Eugène Guye has similarly pointed out, the day when the vital will be reduced to the physico-chemical, the latter will be enriched by properties as yet still unknown (and contemporary molecular biology brings us closer to verifying this twofold prediction). But, however profound Boutroux's thesis may thus be from an epistemological point of view, it is only too clear that his intention to defend moral freedom against dogmatic materialism ends in a refutation of the latter, but does not give to philosophy a specific mode of knowledge (as Bergson, who accepted Boutroux's views, concluded). His critique of science in fact consisted in a conscious realization of the very processes of constructive deduction characteristic of scientific explanation, processes that materialism had not at all perceived.

On the other hand, the earlier no less famous work of Lachelier on *Les fondements de l'induction*, which Lalande shrewdly described as "this little book which one has often had more occasion to admire than to use," certainly contains suggestive remarks on inductive method but endeavors to combine it with a general harmony of nature, implying finality. If this conclusion has been appealed to as a sign of a philosophical knowledge transcending scientific knowledge, one could easily reply that for the scientist induction certainly presupposes an hypothesis, therefore an intention, a plan, etc., but that it is just as successful, with respect to the facts it tries to explain, when these facts involve as large an element as one might wish of randomness, as it is in the case of an organized structure in biology. Computational methods are even more readily available in the first case, as thermodynamics and microphysics demonstrate.

The reaction of philosophers against dogmatic materialism undoubtedly forms one of the factors explaining psychologically the need for a specific mode of suprascientific knowledge. If this reaction has, moreover, met with an easy success, this does not at all prove the originality of the modes of knowledge employed. They have led to either very dubious theses as in J. Lachelier's case, or to an adjustment of epistemology to the realist tendencies of science in opposition to metaphysical scientists and to positivist epistemology.

3. The third factor, which naturally converges with the opposition to materialism but which is much more general, is the desire to give to the coordination of values and to rational faith a mode of knowledge independent of science and transcending it.[1] As an example of this general factor, we may quote the metaphysical psychology of Maine de Biran, one of the sources of the idealistic tendency which has been transmitted from Ravaisson to Lachelier, Boutroux, and Bergson, and which is reflected

---

1 This transcendence being in particular suggested or reinforced by the religious distinction between nature and transcendent realities.

in the eclecticism of V. Cousin and Royer-Collard. Maine de Biran's chief concern was to refute empiricism, and particularly Hume's interpretation of causality, in finding in the self and voluntary effort the direct awareness of substance, force, and causality. In Chapter Four we will return to the errors of introspection that have led to these results and which are a good example of the possible vagaries of an exclusive reference to introspection in opposition to the psycho-physiological, pyscho-pathological and genetic methods. This does not at all mean that these methods neglect the study of consciousness or the subject as such, as the supporters of philosophical psychology believe in stressing the ambiguity of introspection restricted to the "self" and of conscious realization as occurring within the context of conduct. Let us for the moment merely note that, between the ideal of a metaphysical knowledge based directly upon the intuition of the self and its powers and the ideal of a metaphysical knowledge based upon a critique of science, there is only in common the dream of a metaphysical knowledge "superior" to that of science. Apart from this common aim, the two positions are contradictory as the genius of Kant had seen, in his critique of "rational psychology" (that of C. Wolff who shared with Maine de Biran the same Leibnizian inspiration). Such a critique of science consists, in effect, in showing that all experience is a structuring of reality in which the epistemological subject takes an active part, of such a sort that knowledge appears as an interaction between the structuring operations of the subject and the properties of the object. Put in this way there is not the least reason, apart from an affective one, for supposing that "internal experience" is an exception to the common rule, since in introspection a part of the self observes the other part and constitutes therefore a knowing subject in relation to the subject known or to be known. To claim that in introspection there is no such division and that the knowing or epistemological subject is identical with the individual or known subject, would be at one and the same time to deny introspection (for when the two parts of the subject come together again there is no longer introspection, but some activity or other) and to deny the universality as well as the necessary activity of the epistemological subject. This is why Kant has shown that the "self" was not a substance, a force, or a cause, but owed its identity to an internal "unity of apperception." The metaphysical psychology of Maine de Biran (alongside an excellent psychological terminology) therefore transforms the noetic structuring of the known self by the knowing self into a metaphysical self on a more modest plane but in a manner very like that which Fichte, Schelling, Hegel in part, and Schopenhauer were victims of when they based themselves on the Kantian a priori, in order to reconstruct improperly the metaphysical notions of the absolute self.

4. A fourth factor already very noticeable among these great German thinkers, and which has only become worse since then, is that of romanticism, directed increasingly toward irrationalism. From the time that science has pursued an ideal of rationality and metaphysics proposed as its aim the attainment of the whole of reality, there ought therefore to exist, if metaphysics wishes to remain on a higher level than science, a mode of knowledge attaining the irrational itself. Such is intuition in the trans-rational sense, which it has had from Schelling to Bergson. And as such it is an important factor in contemporary existentialism, whose vogue after the Second World War has replaced that of Bergsonism after the First. Kierkegaard, who was of an independent mind, did not like philosophies and rightly found that his own existence was unique and did not fit into the framework of a system. It is true that at a later date the same thing has been done to him as was done to Kant and he has been made the starting point of new systems!

But existence is one thing and knowledge of existence another. If the philosopher does not wish to be mistaken for a novelist, whose peculiar genius is to depict reality through his vision of the world without looking for that which is independent of it (even if he belongs to a realist or naturalist school of philosophy, which is a particular form of personal vision), he will then need to acquire an epistemology of the knowledge of existence. This he will do by asserting that this vision of the world is a knowledge like any other, provided that thinking is kept to a *minimum* and we grasp that which is "offered" in immediately lived experience before all reflection, as if this were a primordial intuition, the source of (or of all) knowledge. We will in Chapter Four return to the fundamental psychological illusion that consists in looking for an absolute beginning in an elementary conscious realization, when all knowledge is connected with action and is therefore conditioned by the earlier schemes of activity; and we shall later in this chapter examine critically Husserl's epistemology. For the moment, we merely need to note that if this intuition of lived experience is given as a philosophical mode of knowledge on a higher level than scientific knowledge, because as Merleau-Ponty said, "The whole universe of science is constructed on the lived world," the metaphysical ambition becomes truly modest and increasingly diverges, together with such an irrationalism (we speak of Merleau-Ponty, for Husserl in the main goes beyond the position originating from him), from the possibility of basing science on it and consequently holding sway over it. In fact, if the world of science is really "constructed" on the lived world, it is not in the manner of an edifice constructed on its foundations, for the aim of scientific thought is always to get further away from this lived world, contradicting it instead of utilizing it. On the other hand, the true starting point of the universe of science is to be looked for in the world of action and not in perception abstracted from its motor and practical context, for the thought operation extends action by simply correcting instead of contradicting it.

5. A final factor essential to the belief in a distinct philosophical mode of knowledge and hence on a higher level than that of scientific knowledge is more commonplace, because it is of a sociological nature, but nevertheless plays an important part not among philosophers themselves but in the ordinary man's attitude toward philosophy. As philosophy has now become a widespread profession, respected and confined within a

Faculty increasingly alien by force of circumstances to that of science, the direct initiation into this discipline, without any preliminary scientific training except at the level of the second degree, leads to habits of thought that foster the belief in a radical independence of philosophical knowledge. The absence of all opposition excludes all verification, and the philosophy of science appears as a simple specialization among all other possible ones. One needs an uncommon philosophical courage to specify with respect to positive knowledge the preliminary epistemological conditions of philosophical reflection. It is too easy, on the contrary, to entertain the illusion of an absolute starting point characteristic of speculation.

On the whole these different reasons converge to produce a common belief in a fundamental dualism of knowledge. On the one hand, "positive" knowledge, of which it is then a question of fixing boundaries, and we will see (from C below onward) the variations of methods as far as this fixing of boundaries is concerned; on the other, an essentially higher kind of knowledge, either offered as the foundation of scientific knowledge or as it concerns other domains in which science is unqualified. The problem we now have to examine, taking as the object of our discussion Bergsonian intuition and phenomenological intuition (not only because they are the product of the two most distinguished parascientific tendencies that have been put forward during this century, but because their authors have themselves been closely in touch with scientific problems), is the analysis of the validity of such modes of knowledge. An intuition being at one and the same time the grasping of an object and the guarantee of truth for the subject, does this duality in unity effectively give a distinct knowledge of experience and deduction, or is the proposed unity only apparent?

(C) The ideal of a suprascientific knowledge originating in the nineteenth century had its beginnings either in the frankly speculative form of German idealism, or in the more modest and more cautious form of epistemology, of a critique of science. This second form has resulted, toward the end of the nineteenth and during the twentieth century, in a new philosophical approach, namely that in the field of "things" and phenomena there was room, alongside scientific knowledge and provided that these limits were specified with sufficient rigor, for another kind of knowledge of these objects and phenomena which would be completely independent and admit of an indefinite progress. Bergson and Husserl have accepted this new approach, but have used two very different methods. The first starts from the antithesis to be found within reality itself, in order to show that, if rational knowledge legitimately succeeds in one of two possible directions, the other remains open to a different mode of knowledge. The second, on the contrary, proceeds by levels in depth, endeavoring to separate out from beneath the spatio-temporal level or "world," but for the same objects and in the same domains, a universe of essences obtained by reductions or "bracketing" in going beneath the initial level. Although pursuing the same aims of limiting scientific knowledge and constituting a specific and autonomous form of philosophical knowledge, the two methods do not therefore overlap, since the positive "world" from which Husserl wishes to escape includes time, while one of the fundamental antitheses of Bergsonism is that of space, the preserve of natural science, and pure duration, the domain of metaphysical intuition. Further, J. P. Sartre, who continues the Husserlian tradition, has said that Bergsonian intuition does not attain being as Husserl's does and that pure duration is only a contingent fact, empirically verified.

It is interesting to note from the start these contradictions between the two main systems based on the philosophical intuition of being, for the two methods proceeding by antithesis or by levels would have been able to be complementary, since they involve similar problems such as the position of mathematics or psychology in relation to philosophical thought. When in the deductive sciences one and the same domain is explored by very different paths, which often occurs, the distinct results are always not only compatible but are able sooner or later to be deduced from each other. In the case of the parascientific intuitions we are going to discuss, one has rather the impression that all the possibilities are tried out in turn because of dissatisfaction with the preceding ones, of such a kind that we need to ask for each system and both together whether, in the field they have each selected, their critique of science still applies today and warrants this metaphysical transcendence in the form they have each hoped for and of which the only common element is this desire for a specific and autonomous form of philosophical knowledge.

The Bergsonian antitheses—living organization and matter, instinct and intelligence, time and space, internal life and action or language, etc.—raise two problems: are they in fact antithetical? Do they converge by overlappings or simple equivalences, or do they exhibit intersections according to all combinations? It is on the solution of these two problems that in the last resort depends the validity of "intuition" put forward as the specific form of philosophical knowledge.

1. The antithesis of organic life and matter is the answer to an evident scientific problem: that of the opposition between the increasing organization that characterizes life and the progressive disorder of a random nature which is the increase in entropy. Further, eminent scientists like Helmholtz, and more recently C. Eugène Guye, have asked if vital mechanisms obey the second law of thermodynamics and whether, on the contrary, we do not need to see in their functioning an anti-randomness that enables them to be independent of it. This dualism, which up to now has simply remained a possibility, has recently been restudied in detail by Bertalanffy and Prigogine in their theory of open systems, whose thermodynamical restatement is, however, still under discussion. Bergsonism can certainly justify its fundamental antithesis by referring to such developments, and the physicist O. Costa de Beauregard, in a philosophical work on *Le Temps* in which he combines precise physics with a somewhat risky metaphysics, has no hesitation in combining the two kinds of concepts of Bergsonism and negative entropy in its twofold sense, physical and informational (as is well

known the concept of entropy plays a central role in information theory).

But if good arguments for the Bergsonian antithesis of life
and matter can therefore be found in the precise field of the
thermodynamics of open and closed systems, where can one find
a justification of the fine picture of the ascending vital stream of
which a part constantly falls back into matter? It is not clear,
even if this dualism is confirmed later on, that it can as such be
generalized to cover the whole of the relationships between life
and matter.

We touch here on the problem of vitalism and of physico-
chemical explanations of vital processes, and with it a question
of method of great interest for our purpose, which is that of the
intervention of philosophers in the different possible scientific
solutions. In the perspective of superimposed levels, which is
that of Husserl, the philosopher does not, in principle, encroach
on the field of the different sciences. Husserl leaves them alone,
recognizing the validity of their methods (even in experimental
psychology) because he is familiar with them. Sartre treats them
with contempt because he is less well acquainted with them,
and he restricts himself to showing that other levels exist where
philosophy is supreme in its apprehension of essences. It is true
that in some cases, for example, in mathematics and physics,
Husserl adds that the scientist himself would have to attain, or
use without realizing it, this intuition of essences and that elsewhere, as in psychology, he wishes to limit the domain of experimental psychology to a restricted field like the spatio-
temporal, and to complete this limited field of study by means
of a philosophical psychology as a necessary supplement. But
the philosopher does not encroach on the field of psychological
knowledge itself. On the contrary, in the perspective of the
Bergsonian antitheses, which has the merit of leaving a larger
field for the sciences, the philosopher concerns himself with
their very solutions, and this raises other problems. For example,
we will see in Chapter Five how Bergson, embarrassed to find
some of the essential characteristics of Bergsonian time in the

theory of relativity when he wished to reserve them for consciousness and life, has oddly enough undertaken to refute Einsteinian mechanics out of hand. In the field of biology, which interests us here, he has naturally taken the side of vitalism against physico-chemical interpretations, since on every question he was concerned to maintain the antithesis of life and matter.

Putting on one side questions of competency and that rule of technicality which F. Gonseth includes among the fundamental principles of his philosophy of science, the danger of such an approach is that it plainly makes a metaphysical truth (which one wishes to be independent) dependent on the theories of the day or on the position of problems relative to the knowledge of the day. In 1907, the date on which L'évolution créatrice appeared, only two solutions seemed possible: the reduction of life to a physico-chemistry conceived as definitive, for the revolutionary changes due to relativity theory and quantum physics had not yet shaken the belief in the apparently immutable structure of classical mechanics and of the physics of Principia; or, on the contrary, a specific theory of vital phenomena bringing up to date classical vitalism in the light of new facts inexplicable by the physico-chemistry then known. It therefore appeared reasonable to side with vitalism, at first because of the notorious inadequacy of mechanistic explanations of that time and, on the other hand, because of the revival of vitalism and particularly of the sensational conversion of Driesch. After having discovered the regeneration of the embryos of sea-urchins divided into two at the blastula stage, Driesch, instead of realizing that he had opened up the new science of causal embryology, which has made so much progress since then, was so impressed by the novelty of this fact that he abandoned any attempt at scientific explanation by appealing to the entelechies of Aristotle so well that he ended his career as a professor of philosophy.

But since then three fundamental events have occurred. The first is the radical transformation of physics, which, without rejecting these earlier achievements, has placed them on a certain level, in adopting for the higher levels (relativity) or lower (microphysics) modes of explanation completely unforeseen until then. It follows from this new flexibility that if one arrives at a physico-chemical explanation of life, it will be by once again enriching physics and thus attaining a reciprocal assimilation and not a one-way reduction. But however satisfactory might be an interpretation respecting the properties of organization constantly stressed by vitalism (and judged by it as inexplicable), it would nonetheless produce the Bergsonian antithesis, since there would be continuity and no longer a radical dualism.

In the second place, this hope of continuity has made real progress with the new discipline of contemporary molecular biology and with the important extensions of biochemistry. In particular, forms of organization have been discovered halfway between physics and living phenomena that possess certain general biological properties like assimilation, and not others like respiration.

In the third place, and this ought to be of particular interest to the philosopher, we have for some years ceased to be faced by the classical alternatives of mechanism or vitalism, chance or finality, etc., because of conceptions of a third type such as the organicism of Bertalanffy, and especially cybernetics, which lies exactly halfway between physics and living phenomena,[2] which enable us today, by means of models of a strictly causal order, to take account of specific properties of the organism: regulations of a finalist appearance, equilibrium, etc. This third perspective, which has arisen as always when one is faced with insoluble alternatives, is certainly the most telling answer to the Bergsonian antitheses. At first because the very terms of the problem seem thus surpassed, but then because the mode of cybernetic thought and the construction of mechanical models simulating finality, learning and even development by levels of equilibrium, constitute a disquieting denial of that congenital

---

[2] See the interesting interpretations that C. H. Waddington, among others, derives from it, which thus end in a kind of *tertium* between Lamarckism and Neo-Darwinism.

maladaptation of intelligence to the living realities, which another thesis of Bergson asserts (see under 3).

2. The antithesis of the lived duration (as far as the organism or the psychological subject are concerned) and physical space is much weaker because here Bergson—who had at first specialized in the field of mathematical and physical knowledge and then went on to study psychology but merely by using the method of introspection—sins both by misunderstanding the psychogenetic data and by obvious error in the field of physics.

As far as the psychogenetic data are concerned (we will return to this in Chapter Four from the point of view of the critique of philosophical psychology and only discuss it here from the epistemological point of view), the Bergsonian duration with its property of neither being metrical nor spatialized, but admitting of dilation or contraction according to its content and consisting in this self-same content as long as construction or creation continues ("time is invention or it is nothing at all"), is only one of the aspects of lived time. And yet it is an aspect that is not "purely" temporal, for if lived time is invention it is still the case that this construction of which time is the "stuff" ("time is the very stuff of reality") flows with a velocity which is neither null nor infinite. Time therefore presupposes passage, that of the perceived external processes or of the internal mental processes, and this is a first important point that the psychogenetic study of time seems to reveal. At a later date, the subject spontaneously arrives at three sorts of temporal operations that partially structure this lived time independently of all physical knowledge: (a) a seriation of events according to an order of succession; (b) an overlapping of intervals such that for the ordered events ABC . . . (internal or external events), the duration AB is judged to be shorter than AC even if these times are not homogeneous as far as uniform passage is concerned; (c) a metric resulting from the synthesis of the two, such that if duration AB extends over BC, this entails AC = 2AB. This metric presupposes neither an external clock nor a reference to physics, and Bergson, who is fond of musical imagery, should have remembered that the most popular and spontaneous music presupposes such a metric (independently even of the musical notation in minims, crochets, and quavers). The lived duration of the child is thus at first pre-operational or intuitive, then partially operational, and that of the adult still shares in both.

As for physics, Bergson regards its conception of time as completely spatialized and no longer related to this lived duration. He had not seen that physical time is itself also relative to velocity (which was understandable before relativity but at least shows that philosophical knowledge had not anticipated the latter). From his concept of a time spatialized and so to speak emptied of its content, Bergson has then drawn this conclusion, which has appeared to him as a confirmation of his theses: that in varying all the velocities in the universe, we would not at all change any of the temporal relations measured by the physicist. There then occurred the unexpected discovery of relativity, which contradicted this thesis: whence Bergson's attempt to refute Einstein and A. Metz's answer showing the errors in Bergson's reasoning.

Nothing remains therefore of the antithesis of the lived duration and of spatialized time or physical space. Physical space is itself also relative to its content and both depend on velocity. As for the relations between this antithesis and that of life and matter, it is clear that the evolution of life is an historical development which presupposes a continual temporal "invention" (without doubt even having periods of acceleration and deceleration). But life is just as much spatial invention, for the unbelievable diversity of forms presupposes a remarkable geometrical combinatorial system. It has been shown that the passage from the fish or shell form to the closely related phylogenetic forms involves well-defined geometrical transformations, topological varieties, affine, etc.

3. We now come to the central antithesis of intelligence and instinct, central from the epistemological point of view, since Bergson deems that intelligence only adequately understands matter and space, while instinct, alone or extended into

intuition, is the sole mode of knowledge adapted to life and "pure" duration.

The ideas of Bergson on instinct were prompted by those of Fabre, an excellent observer but whose interpretations were somewhat influenced by his theology: immutability of instinct, as opposed to the flexibility of intelligence, knowledge infinitely precise but limited and blind, in opposition to trial and error, but also to consciousness and intelligence, etc. However, since then our knowledge about intelligence itself as about instinct has been greatly increased by psychogenetic data for the former, and by experimental studies for the latter, of the so-called objectivist school (Tinbergen, Lorenz, von Holst, etc.) and of the French school of Grassé, Delaurence, etc., and the problem is no longer stated in the same terms.

In order to formulate it adequately, it is necessary at first to note that it would be wrong to confine oneself to the alternatives continuity or discontinuity stated in linear terms, as if intelligence developed linearly on one and the same level. In reality, intelligence is constructed by successive stages of equilibrium, such that the activity begins on each stage by a reconstruction of that which was already acquired in the preceding stage, but under a more restricted form. Thus, one observes in the child a first stage of intelligence, before language, under a sensori-motor form but which already takes us sufficiently far: schemes of conservation with the construction of the permanent object, reversibility with the practical "group" of displacements, objectified and spatialized causality, etc. At the following stage, which is that of representative thought and of concrete operations, that which has been acquired on a sensori-motor level needs to be completely reconstructed on the plane of representation (which covers the period two-six years) before the formation toward seven years of age of the first representative conservations and the first reversible operations. Then, toward eleven to twelve years, a third stage characterized by formal or hypothetico-deductive operations, begins by a restructuring of the concrete operations so that the new operations can be constituted as second-order operations integrating the earlier ones.

If intelligence itself thus develops in a nonlinear manner by successive constructions on different levels, then the lower, or sensori-motor, level cannot be regarded as absolute and ought to be rooted in an earlier stage of an organic nature, which would then be constituted by the system of reflexes and instincts. There is no difference in nature between reflexes and instincts, the first only consists of differentiations starting from the more global rhythmic activities.

On the other hand, as far as instinct is concerned it is now known that neither its infallibility nor its immutability is absolute, and one finds in certain cases (Delaurence) a small capacity for learning which seems to merge into intelligence. What has been further established—and this is fundamental—is the existence of hereditary "meaningful signs" that release motor activity. These signs are recognized by assimilation and assimilatory schemes (quite different from mechanical associations), are generalizable (all sorts of "decoys" can be constructed that imitate the natural sign and which show the degree of generalization), and above all sometimes relatively flexible. In the case of the *stigmergies* of Grassé, in which termites mold kneaded balls of earth into pillars, the order of succession of operations is not constant but exhibits appreciable variations. Finally—and this is the main point—one finds at all levels, down to the protozoa, learning behavior on the fringe of instinct. In the human young, one can follow by continuous transitions the successive stages proceeding from spontaneous global movements (akin to instinct) and from the reflexes themselves to conditioned conduct, to the first habits, and to acts of intelligence properly so called through the coordination of assimilatory schemes specific to habits.

All these facts seem therefore to lead us toward an interpretation according to which instinct would form a sort of logic of the bodily organs (the logic resulting in a general fashion from the coordination of actions or operations), from which is derived at a higher level the logic of acquired sensori-motor conduct and of sensori-motor intelligence, whose existence is so plain among the anthropoids and the human young.

4. If the preceding antitheses all vanish on analysis, the fundamental epistemological thesis of Bergson becomes considerably weakened. According to this thesis, intelligence is inapt to comprehend life and only adapts itself to space and unorganized matter and, moreover, only to their static and discontinuous aspects.

Bergson's first argument is that intelligence originates from action on matter, but there is a twofold difficulty here. In the first place intelligence arises from action in general and not only from action on matter: on other persons, on (and by means of) one's own body, as well as inanimate objects. In the second place logic and mathematics do not result from the form of the objects to which one can apply them—otherwise we fall back into classical empiricism—but rather from general coordinations of actions (combining, ordering, putting into correspondence, etc.) irrespective of the nature of the objects to which these actions are directed.

The second argument is that intelligence reconstructs the continuous by means of the discontinuous, movement by means of the static, etc., by a method analogous to the "cinematographic process" according to a famous comparison. But on this central point Bergson argues as if intelligence is simply reducible to images, for the mental image is static by nature, inapt to grasp the continuous. Bergson, in fact, completely neglects the existence of *operations*, which essentially concern transformations and not merely mental states, which consist in acts and not in images, and which as such achieve activity and are thus creative of dynamic structures. In his metaphor of the "cinematographic process," Bergson sees only the successive snapshots that correspond therefore to images, but he neglects the motor activity that ensures their development, and it is in this in which intelligence itself resides.

As for the assumed heterogeneity between logico-mathematical intelligence and life in general, two answers can nowadays be given to Bergsonism. This form of intelligence is essentially operational and the fundamental operations derive therefore from the coordinations of actions, a coordination that is already a biological phenomenon, since it is based on neural coordinations (and in this respect one recalls that W. McCulloch and Pitts have found that the synaptic coordinations exhibited all the types of relationships of the "logic of propositions"). But there is more to it. The psychogenetic study of the formation of operations shows that they constitute the final form of equilibrium (the operations are entirely reversible because they are in a state of equilibrium) of a succession of semi-reversible regulations that form its rough outline or preparation. The concepts of regulation and equilibrium are essentially biological. It seems therefore clear that there exists some continuity between the organic self-regulation, which undoubtedly is one of the most important of the biological processes, and that self-regulation, or mental self-correction, which is logic. On the other hand, unless one is an empiricist or an *a priorist* (or Platonist), it is difficult to see how mathematics can apply so admirably to physical reality if the logico-mathematical structures are not deeply rooted in biological organization, which is at once the origin of the subject's activity and the reason for this fundamental applicability.

The second answer to the thesis that there is a heterogeneity between intelligence and life is that the group of organic regulations from which elementary mental operations seem therefore to have sprung, can nowadays be given a logico-mathematical treatment. This is derived not from classical or relativity mechanics, nor from the physics of solid bodies, etc., but rather from cybernetics, the new discipline which can simulate some of the essential aspects of "living" things. Ashby's homeostat shows how the problems can be solved by an all or none equilibrium, the "perceptron" of Rosenblith how an organism can learn something, the "genetron" of Papert how development can take place by successive stages of equilibrium. In a general fashion models using loops or *feedback* give a possible explanation of regulations and are even able to give us what is referred to today as "mechanical equivalents of finality." It is therefore no longer possible to consider operational intelligence as being forever blind as far as living processes are concerned.

5. From these many antitheses of which there remains little today, Bergson has finally derived his central thesis of a metaphysical knowledge *sui generis* and irreducible to reason or scientific knowledge. Such would be intuition, or instinct, becoming conscious of itself and attaining directly the realities peculiar to life that would be pure duration of the creative activity of consciousness. Bergson, who was constantly looking for reality, told us how to attain this intuition of the vital: to introspect one's consciousness in throwing off the superficial and resistant features constituted by habits due to action on matter, to language, and social life; to delve deeply into oneself until one reaches regions close to that of dreams or the creative unconscious, and to discover in these depths the *élan vital* as it surges forth in its spirituality and in its becoming.

It has often been remarked that this personal intuition of Bergson was very much the product of a refined intelligence for which reflection did not claim to attain the goal directly, but began by selecting, isolating, and abstracting in order to reconstruct an extremely elaborate model of duration. Sartre reproaches Bergson somewhat rudely for taking pure duration as an empirical fact or a contingent accident. We will make the precisely opposite point in showing that it is really the product of a singularly advanced intellectual construction, and also put the Sartrean introspections in the same category of what could be termed constructed introspections.

Far from being the initial starting point like the Cartesian or Husserlian *Cogito*, from which the various features of the system could be developed, Bergsonian intuition is a resultant of many analyses carried out on a reflective level. It might be said that it has directed them, but it is then as an intellectual intuition, *i.e.* those global hypotheses that we "feel" lead somewhere before we can analyze them out into particular arguments.

We cannot therefore at all see, neither considered as a resultant nor as a guiding hypothesis, in what way it is a question of a *sui generis* mode of knowledge peculiar to metaphysics.

Edouard Le Roy has considered the Bergsonian philosophy as revolutionary in character and has compared it with the Kantian and Socratic revolutions, because both of them had given rise to a method. The difference all the same is that if Bergsonism has had a good deal of influence, it is not due to the application of his "intuition." It is rather because of the emphasis he put on becoming and on the lived duration, moreover at the same time at which the *Données immédiates* appeared, the psychologist W. James just as vigorously rejected associationism in favor of the "stream of consciousness" (see Chapter Four under D). But the creative becoming is neither the justification of intuition nor of metaphysics and one can give the following counter-argument. Brunschvicg had a profound admiration for Bergson (and went so far, so it seemed to me, that he even often imitated without wanting to the way in which Bergson pronounced *t* in the English manner).[3] There was therefore a probable influence here: the growth of thought according to Brunschvicg in mathematical philosophy, physics, or ethics is a creative process, unpredictable and without finality, which is, in a striking fashion, the Bergsonian duration but applied to the history of intelligence.

(D) If the Bergsonian antitheses and oppositions that occur on the plane of reality, studied by science itself, thus run the risk of being contradicted by the advance of the latter, Husserl's method of levels of phenomena with its "reductions" and

[3] This book being something of a confession, I cannot resist the pleasure of recalling a visit I paid Bergson when, many years ago, I gave my first paper to the *Société française de Philosophie*. I was very thrilled to see the great Bergson but, after the influence he had had on me during adolescence, I had difficulty in realizing that the old gentleman facing me, kept indoors by his rheumatism, was the same Bergson whose writings I had read so much formerly: "You have," he said to me kindly, "introduced discontinuities between the child and the adult. I am myself rather in favor of continuity." "Yes," I replied with feeling, "I know. . . ." I stopped myself just in time: I was going to say, "How Bergsonian you are!"

"bracketing" does not involve the same danger, since it does not contradict science and only seeks to complement it by a mode of knowledge specifically metaphysical. But it runs the complementary risk of seeing these levels, seemingly isolated and self-contained, encroached upon by scientific analysis in its inevitable advance.

The great merit of the Husserlian intuitions is that they are related straightaway to the "things themselves," therefore to phenomena, and do not start from the dualism of subject and object. Husserl is just as much opposed to idealism or to Kantian *a priorism*, which attributes everything to the subject, as to empiricism or to positivism, which neglects everything in favor of the object. The fundamental datum is therefore for him the phenomenon as an indissociable interaction, and it is from this fact that he wishes to start in order to attain reality. It is through this aspect of its doctrine that phenomenology has influenced Gestalt theory in psychology, which has moved toward a completely anti-Husserlian physicalism by increasingly neglecting the subject, because together with the notion of an indissociable interaction, Gestalt psychology has equally inherited from phenomenology what might be called its actualism or its complete lack of concern for the historical or genetic dimensions.

The interaction between subject and object can be analyzed from two points of view. If we take up the factual point of view, i.e. that of the phenomenon as given without any immediate desire to transcend it, this interaction is a moment of history, history of the individual or history of ideas, therefore psychogenesis or history of science, and our inquiry will consist in retracing the phases of such an interaction. Brunschvicg has often been reproached for his idealism, because he liked the word, and above all because he had neglected biology in his studies in the philosophy of mathematics and physics; but Parodi accused him of positivism in the sense of scientism with neither more nor less justification. In reality Brunschvicg was as much as Husserl an opponent both of empiricism and *a priorism*, and returned just as often to the interaction of the subject and object, which "grip," said he, constantly modifying each other. But he studied these reciprocal modifications in the field of history by the historico-critical method. In the field of genetic psychology I have myself constantly stressed the same interaction, and if I consantly return to the activities of the subject this is because psychologists of an empiricist tendency (everything happens) neglect it too often (which will not prevent some readers of this book from calling me a positivist).

But one can also, in starting from the interaction of the subject and object, or from consciousness in its "relationship to the world," limit oneself to outlining an internal or epistemological analysis, which will then be called "ontological," since it refers just as much to the thing as to the subject intuiting it. This will be Husserl's method, but in order to understand its lacunae as much as its ambitions, hence in its "anti-historicism" as much as in its attempt to grasp the nontemporal essences, we need nevertheless to do a bit of history.

As we have seen in Chapter Two, Husserl began with a fine book on the philosophy of arithmetic in which he tried to take account of numerical operations by certain mental operations, one of which is colligation, or the combination of elements into a whole. This book has been criticized by logicians, who have accussed him of "psychologism," i.e. of proceeding from a fact to a norm, which is certainly inadmissible. In principle, the logicians were undoubtedly right, and Husserl was so convinced of it that he became converted to the cult of nontemporal truths (he had had an excellent mathematical training), and he concentrated on the search for the methods by which the subject X object attains them. But unfortunately for his later doctrine, he has not at this turning point in his career grasped two important things.

The first might appear to be secondary, and it will be said that I speak here as a psychologist, but its importance will be seen later: Husserl would certainly have been able to continue doing good psychology without falling into "psychologism." All that he needed to know was that he studied a "natural" arithmetic without as such claiming to legislate for the logic of numbers, and to construct, moreover, limited logistic models corresponding to what he found and to compare them to the completely abstract models constructed by Frege, Schröder, etc. There would thus have not been any psychologism, qua passage from fact to norm, but an interdisciplinary study of concrete psychological relationships and of formal or abstract logical genealogies. This would at least have prevented him from making at a later date an erroneous critique of psychologism, because he has not seen that one can do precisely what he had failed to do by giving in too easily to logicians unaware of the possibilities of psychology.

The second misunderstanding has had much greater consequences. Husserl was not a professional logician nor one by inclination, since he did not interest himself in formalism as such and he believed in the "things" and in the interaction subject $\times$ object central to phenomena. Having given in to the verdict of the logicians and having therefore renounced all psychologism, he set about discovering how, in starting from this phenomenological interaction, one can attain nontemporal truths. And then convinced of the fact (i.e. the hypothesis) that the psychological subject does not arrive at them by himself, insofar as he is inseparable from a spatio-temporal "world," he has thought of a method of escape or liberation from this natural world so as to attain a deeper level than "mundane" consciousness, and he thus believed he had discovered the possibility of pure or transcendental "intuitions." At the same time, he hoped to open the way for an autonomous philosophical knowledge, freed from the empirical subject and from the sciences connected with it. Husserl's fundamental mistake lies in the fact that his transcendental subject is still a subject and that "pure intuition" is still the activity of a subject (in which the "object," or "essence," admittedly enters in, but if there is intuition there is, nonetheless, a subject): it follows that, "transcendental" or empirical, reference to such an intuition is still psychologism, that is to say, a passage from fact to norm.

The "phenomenological reduction," or the freeing of consciousness from the spatio-temporal world in order to arrive at an intuition of essences, calls then for two sorts of remarks, one of a logical and the other of a psychological order.

From the point of view of logic, the logicians Cavailles and Beth have said all that is necessary. Logic, which is a formal axiomatic system is only grounded on itself, *i.e.* on normative rules that permit the elaboration of a formal system: definitions starting from concepts arbitrarily selected as given and undefined, axioms (or undemonstrated propositions), rules of inference and theories deduced by these rules starting from axioms and definitions. To give an intuitive basis for such systems is to go outside the system in order to explain epistemologically how this is possible, but we do not provide a foundation for this system in providing a guarantee of its validity. This validity is only normative and consists in a guarantee of noncontradiction (which moreover is only obtained in constructing systems of a higher order: see Chapter Two under 5), while for the logician, intuition is only a fact: there is therefore a passage from fact to norm. To say that the intuition is "true" presupposes a normative justification, not given by the intuition itself, being only the expression of the necessity experienced by a subject. As Cavailles said, either logic is dependent upon the intuition of a transcendental subject, and is no longer absolute (which one would like it to be), or it is absolute, and no longer requires a transcendental intuition. And Beth, following Cavailles, concludes like him that for the logician phenomenology is only one psychologism among others, but developed in another language.

From the psychological point of view, our approach will be very different and we will fully sympathize with the central problem stated by Husserl, that of the search for "pure," or nontemporal, concepts, as well as with his "phenomenological reduction," or the freeing of consciousness from the spatiotemporal "world." We shall see in his criticism of psychology only the sign of a disappointed love, for, in remaining on the level of consciousness, of the intuitions of the subject, and above all of his "intentions," he shows that he is not a pure logician. If, on the affective level, a disappointed love cannot generally be cured, on that of ideas, everything in the end becomes a matter of method and of verification. Let us therefore begin with the latter in order then to pass on to the former.

If we are sympathetic to the Husserlian problem of the liberation from the spatio-temporal, this is not due to direct or indirect influence (I had to my shame not read a single line of Husserl until recently, dismayed by what Sartre and Merleau-Ponty had derived from him). It is for a much more decisive reason: any study of the formation and development of concepts and intellectual operations leads to such a problem and enables one to see how this liberation from the spatio-temporal occurs under a spontaneous and directly observable form.

I will only quote as an example (among other more particular cases) the structuring of operations. A logico-mathematical operation is essentially atemporal, and this can be verified, among others, from its reversibility: if $2 + 3 = 5$ then $5 - 3 = 2$ by immediate necessity and independently of the temporal order of the symbols or of individual thought. The fact that the operation can proceed in two directions and that one of them implies the other by immediate logical necessity is sufficient proof that neither of the two is temporal. This operational necessity is only grasped at a later age and constitutes the chief problem for the subject in the formation of his operations. As long as it is not attained there is no possibility of additive composition: the subject of four to five years will think, for example, that if 10 counters are split up into two groups of 4 and 6, that there are more counters in the two groups than in the one and this even if the sum is 10 in each case. The names of numbers only serve to specify the elements but do not at all prescribe the postulate that the whole is equal to the sum of its parts, because this postulate presupposes the operation of addition, which presupposes reversibility. The passage from 10 to $4 + 6$ appears to the subject as an irreversible transformation, which has changed everything including the numerical value of the collection. The operation presupposes reversibility and the latter conservation, etc., in a complete system (a "group," etc.) essentially extratemporal.

The surprising fact is that the behavior of subjects toward seven to eight years conforms to this system and before that (on the average) it does not. How are we to explain this sort of conversion or "phenomenological reduction" in the young child? Let us begin simply by describing it. Psychologically, operations originate from actions: the operation of addition from that of combining. But the actions are in themselves irreversible, and it is insufficient then to internalize them in thought in order to make them reversible. On the other hand, once internalized these actions give rise to "regulations," which are not yet operational, but already involve an approximate reversibility. For example, for a child of five to six years of age, a row of 10 counters placed before him and then spaced out will make more than 10, and if brought closer together will make less than 10 in the absence of reversibility and as a result of the strong influence of the spatial configuration (of the "spatio-temporal" world!). If, however, the elements are increasingly spaced out, he will end up by saying, "There are now less, they are not close enough." These regulations express themselves therefore by compensations which modify or restrain the transformations still irreversible, and these compensations are the sign of a progressive equilibrium the result of which is then the following. At a given moment (and this sometimes happens in front of the experimenter), the child when faced with the division of 10 into 4 and 6, will say, for example: "That makes more. Oh no! you have only separated them and they can be put back. That comes to the same thing. This must be since they are the same, etc." In short, there is an understanding, in general sudden, of reversibility and of the logical necessity it involves.

We deal here, of course, with only one of the phases of the refining of concepts of the formation of operations, and the process only then becomes more marked with the constitution of formal operations divorced still further from their spatio-temporal content. But this phase already raises a problem that relates to that of Husserl: How does the operation become independent of temporal irreversibility? I remember having been so struck by this problem when I came across it for the first time that I started off (it is long ago now, by way of an apology for referring to my youth) by asking if, with operational reversibility, there did not occur almost instantaneous neural transmissions, whose speed greater or equal to that of light would enable time to be reversed or annulled. . . . Then I gave up these wild speculations (I also thought of an anti-random element that would suppress in the thought of the child the increase of entropy connected with the general irreversibility of the individual spontaneous consciousness), and I realized that we were here concerned above all with a question of levels in the activities of the subject. Irreversibility is connected with the consciousness of the individual subject who, restricting himself solely to the action itself and the subjective impressions accompanying it, is carried away by the stream of internal and external events and strongly influenced by the apparent configurations. On the other hand, the discovery of operational reversibility marks the constitution of the epistemological subject, which becomes divorced from action proper so as to concern itself with the general coordinations of action, *i.e.* with those permanent "forms" of combination, overlapping, ordering, correspondence, etc., which relate actions to each other and thus constitute their necessary substructure.

We then see at the start that this change of level in the activities of a subject which, from being an individual subject becomes an epistemological one, through the internal progress of the coordinations of his thought and through an equilibrium that substitutes logical necessity for empirical verification, exhibits some similarities to a phenomenological "reduction." This is, if I have really understood the intentions of a phenomenology that aims to become general, *i.e.* to describe processes common to all subjects and not specific to the consciousness of the philosopher who describes them. These include the phenomenological reduction, the intuition of "essences," or the "intention" that attains the forms which ought to characterize all scientific thought in the scientist himself if not obscured by his positivism, or in the pre-scientific subject constructing the concepts that will form the starting point for scientific thought. In this case the psychogenetic facts just noted would constitute a simple confirmation of phenomenology, and it is thus that some followers of the school, like Aron Gurwitsch and others, understand it.

We need, in fact, to emphasize strongly the convergence between that which the psychology of intelligence studies under the name of operational "structures" and that which Husserl's phenomenology seeks to reach below the level of empirical or spatio-temporal consciousness. The notion of "structure" is not at all reducible to a simple formalization due to the observer's mind: it expresses, on the contrary, through its formalizations to which, moreover, it lends itself, properties constitutive of the structured "being." It plays therefore, but in a field open to verification and deductive inference, the role one would wish to give to "eidetic" knowledge: being at once accessible to the observer and a profounder reality than the phenomenal existence for which it provides the justification. It completely fulfills the function which one expects from "essences," with this difference, which is in its favor, that it is rigorously deduced instead of only being intuited, or if one prefers it, that its intuition condenses or summarizes a deductive synthesis instead of letting it slip.

But we then need to raise the question of methods and ask if the disappointed love of Husserl for psychology has not led him, as happens in such a case, to some unfairness and lack of understanding that has become systematic. Let us first recall that any problem can become scientific if it is sufficiently delimited and admits of a solution verifiable by everyone. There is not therefore a fixed boundary between science and philosophy, the boundary being a variable one and a function of the position of the problems and of the state of the verifications. From this it follows that the boundaries proposed by positivist philosophy or by any other philosophy remain arbitrary and subject to modification according to the state of knowledge. Husserl, having abandoned psychology in order to search for extratemporal realities, has believed it necessary, while recognizing fully and explicitly (*Ideen*) the legitimacy of an experimental psychology as a "natural" science, to assign limits to it. This psychology is, according to him, restricted to the spatiotemporal world and consequently other methods are necessary to go beyond it.

The great shortcoming of phenomenology is its neglect of historical and genetic points of view (it does nowadays speak of a transcendental genesis, but somewhat belatedly and on another level). Taking up the perspective of an absolute beginning of knowledge, characteristic of the *Cogito*, it has had no difficulty in digging in depth, starting from actual adult consciousness, in order to find below the spatio-temporal level, levels obtained by reduction or bracketing, such that spatio-temporal psychology has no longer any concern there: when the apparent realization of the dream of a mode of knowledge and of a psychology both specifically philosophical. But as soon as the historical or genetic perspective is reintroduced, we are then faced with the following difficulty: in studying the child from birth to seven to eight years, we are engaged in scientific psychology, since the subject is then strongly influenced by the spatio-temporal universe in his conceptions of number, of logical class (classifications in terms of shape), and in his pre-operational reversibility. But when toward seven to eight years there occurs a first "reduction" leading to operational reversibility and to the first forms of atemporal necessity, ought the "scientific" psychologist pack his bags and leave the field free to philosophers? Or ought he himself become a phenomenologist?

Labels being entirely secondary, the only question—but it is a serious one—is that of the methods of discovery and invention: intuitions (eidetic, "intentional," etc.) or observation and experiment. If science is open-ended, it would be unable to formulate a priori any objection against the existence of eidetic intuitions. I see no difficulty if one thus wishes to describe the progress of thought which results from the decentrations in relation to the individual subject and which marks the appearance by stages of the epistemological subject, at seven years, at twelve years, at twenty years, or at fifty years. But what the psychologist, mindful of verification, asks is simply that the subject studying this intuition should not always be the same as that which experiences it. In other words, I have confidence in what I observe in a child of seven or twelve years (from the time of the formation of elementary operations, then formal ones), because, if I am unsure as to what is going on in one subject I can observe another, etc., and that, after a hundred, I have sufficient cases to make all the cross-checkings and tests I need. But if I observe in myself "intuitions" that I experience, from the first I only observe the already elaborated, instead of observing the process of formation; and then what I see is so bound up with my conception of it and so dependent on my intentions of finding this or that, that it becomes utterly impossible to trace with certainty the boundary between the "intuitions" of the introspector and that of the introspected. And finally, I fear that this difference between "eidetic analysis" practiced on oneself and the analysis pure and simple of thought in its formation and in its functioning is the only reason that makes the first "philosophical" and not the second (we shall return to this in Chapter Four).

In short, phenomenological problems as much as one wishes, but not the phenomenological method, not as long as it remains confined to the philosopher's consciousness, and we now have to see why.

(E) From the present standpoint, the only two modes of knowledge which can appear specific to philosophy and alien or superior to scientific knowledge are intuition and the dialectic. We need therefore to examine them closely.

Scientific knowledge comprises two fundamental modes: experimental interpretation and algorithmic deduction; they can moreover both be according to the case more or less static or

I

dialectic. In short, the sciences presuppose facts and norms, and they are concerned with discovering or elaborating them both.

The surprising character of philosophical intuition, as conceived by Bergson and Husserl in spite of their fundamental differences, is that they wish to combine both fact and norm into a single whole, instead of combining them in diverse ways as is the case in the many kinds of scientific discipline. The problem is then to see whether this union is fertile or whether its product is a mongrel one or a sterile hybrid.

Eidetic intuition ought to be able to give the scientist himself, Husserl tells us, knowledge of the essences he uses, if his positivism has not made him short-sighted. A science in which one has clasically spoken of intuition and of logical or normative necessity, and which, moreover, has remained unaffected (no more than others in this respect) by positivist fiats is geometry, where it may be of interest to see what has become of "intuition" over the centuries. A Husserlian purist will perhaps answer that as geometry concerns itself with space, it arises therefore from the spatio-temporal world and not from "pure" essences. But geometrical space has so affected the problem of essences that Plato has derived his intuition of *Ideas* from it.

The geometrical intuition of the Greeks, therefore, fully conforms with what we have just said about philosophical intuition, insofar as it is a combination of norm and fact. Euclid has, indeed, only selected intuitive axioms, in opposition to modern axiomatics of which the axioms are arbitrarily selected provided that they are all necessary, together sufficient and independent. These intuitive axioms of Euclid involve the two characteristics of norm and fact: they are on the one hand, self-evident, which is guaranteed by their normative truth, and, on the other, applicable to all geometrical forms in the real world, which guarantees their "relationship to the object" or applicability to fact.

In recent times, on the other hand, and before the present period (from the time of Hilbert and Einstein, among others), geometrical intuition has suffered a series of crises that it would take too long to go into, but whose general tendency is sufficiently clear: it is that of a progressive separation of norm and fact. With the Cartesian dualism of thought and extension, the latter, although "clear and distinct," is nonetheless directed toward facts, but it derives from thought its normative justification with analytical geometry, among others. In Kant, space is straightforwardly a form of sensibility and not of the understanding, and nineteenth-century mathematicians tended to regard geometry as a form of applied mathematics, as opposed to pure mathematics: algebra, analysis and the theory of numbers. However, the discovery of non-Euclidean geometrics and the structuring of geometrics according to the abstract forms of the theory of groups (from Sophus Lie, etc., to the Erlangen program of F. Klein) strongly maintained the tendency to a logical and normative elaboration of geometrical intuition. The break finally occurred with the contemporary period and geometrical intuition, while remaining important from the heuristic point of view, has lost its value as a form of knowledge and truth in favor of these two components henceforth disjoined. On the one hand, a logical geometry, which no longer has anything intuitive about it (as far as the demonstrations are concerned) and reduced to pure formalizable axiomatic systems (with the unification of topology and algebra, etc.); on the other hand, a geometrical physics, like that of Einstein, which studies the space of physical objects and no longer that of thought.

The lesson of this historical development is therefore that the initial intuition, which is at once both fact and norm, is complex and not a necessary cognitive unity, and that, in its development, its two components have had to separate out. It is, then, not only proper but also necessary to ask if philosophical intuition is not a *forteriori* of a similar complex nature and open to the same dangers, *i.e.* separating out inevitably into the two sorts of components: some psychological and physical and others logical or normative.

The interesting feature of intuition according to Husserl, which allows him to believe its components to be indissociable, is that it is based on an interaction that is indissociable, that of subject and object, creative of "phenomena." But, and it is this from which the sophism proceeds, it is one thing to say that the *phenomenon* results from an indissociable bond between subject and object and another to say that the *intuition* of the phenomenon and all that one undertakes to find there involves an indissociable bond between the normative elements of the subject and the factual elements relative to the object. In reality the phenomenon "being what it is," its intuition remains subject to error as to truth, as do all the activities of the subject. And to say that the phenomenon is internal to consciousness, and that it is primitive, immediate, etc., changes nothing at all, for a primitive datum can be less true and more deceptive than an elaborated one, because of the twofold meaning of the term "subjective" (distorting or knowing). The belief according to which intuition is at one and the same time "contact with the object" and "true," requires therefore a twofold proof, from fact and normative justification; as soon as one looks for these proofs, intuition separates into experiment and deduction.

Such is equally the fate of other concepts belonging to phenomenological intuitionism. An "essence" is both a concept of the subject and the phenomenal nucleus of the object. But how are we to know if the essence is "true" without examining separately the experience of the object (while submitting it, of course, to the epistemological critique) and also the logic used by the subject to elaborate his concepts? "Intention" is a directing of the subject's consciousness toward essences and productive of cognitive forms, but if it is necessary to recall constantly the way consciousness is thus directed, intention will not suffice either in spite of Thomism, to ensure a necessary success, and this even on the phenomenal level. For the hell of knowledge, like that of other sinners who are not philosophers, is also paved with good "intentions."

It will be said that by separating intuition into experimental verification and deduction, we dissociate the interaction of the subject and object, acknowledged as indissociable. This is not the case: but we replace as the analysis of the phenomenon itself requires, the idea, completely arbitrary today, of an absolute beginning, by the dialectical idea of a constant becoming. The history of science as much as the study of individual development shows that this interaction, while remaining indissociable, passes from an undifferentiated phase to one of coordination. Starting from a state of centration on a self uncognizant of itself and in which the subjective and objective are inextricably intermingled, the progressive decentration of the subject leads to a twofold movement, of externalization, tending to physical objectivity, and internalization tending to logico-mathematical coherence. But physical knowledge remains impossible without the logico-mathematical framework and it is impossible to construct the latter without its being applicable to "any" object whatever. It is this twofold movement that intuitionism neglects, and this is why "intuition" remains an extremely poor method for philosophical knowledge.

(F) The problem of dialectical knowledge is an entirely different one, and, if we have spoken little of it, this is because few writers, since Hamelin, make of it a method of knowledge specific to philosophy. Indeed, the mode of dialectical thought is so inherent in all the sciences involving an evolution or a becoming that every dialectical epistemology necessarily bases itself on experience acquired in such disciplines, social or natural.

However, the conversion of Sartre to dialectical thought as well as the way one or two East European philosophers are thinking shows the possibility of a separation into two dialectics. One imperialist in character and claiming to guide science, the other immanent in the spontaneous developments of science and crystallized on a conceptual level into a more general epistemology. The first is the dialectic of concepts, which plays a leading part in Hegel's philosophy and is ready to reappear in other forms in all situations where philosophy takes up again its ambition of being the guardian of absolute knowledge. In his *Critique de la raison dialectique*, Sartre explains that true explanation ought to be constructive in opposition to the inductive generalizations described by positivism and he seems confident of the actual extension of constructivism to all scientific domains, experimental as well as deductive. The second form of dialectic is not concerned with concepts as such, but with interpretations of experiential data and thus corresponds at the present time to one of the most vital tendencies of the philosophy of science, in its specialized epistemologies. This is not, however, the place to discuss it, for the radical opposition between such a dialectic and all "intuition" is sufficiently clear.

To summarize Chapters Two and Three, we can, it seems, conclude as follows. The metaphysical function proper to philosophy ends in a wisdom and not a mode of knowledge because it is a rational coordination of all values, including cognitive values, but transcends them without remaining on the plane of knowledge. On the other hand, and without exaggeration, it can be maintained that all that has been produced of value by philosophers in the field of knowledge itself, and the last thing in the world we would dream of doing is to dispute its immense importance, has been either due to a reflection on sciences already constituted or in process of constitution, or to fruitful suggestions anticipating the possibility of sciences yet to be constituted, of which the history of ideas has given subsequent proof. As against this, the only mode of knowledge appealed to as the specific method proper to philosophy, namely intuition, appears to be complex. Its analysis reveals two components as yet undifferentiated—experiment and deductive inference.

But how are we to explain this confidence in the diverse forms of intuition, which is thus the chief illusion of philosophies claiming to attain a suprascientific form of knowledge? From the fact that there exists a group of vital values, whose axiological evaluation transcends the bounds of scientific knowledge, and from the fact that these values correspond, moreover, to specific intuitions, alien to the knowledge of being but constitutive of such values precisely insofar as they are vital, one concludes that these intuitive methods, perfectly legitimate as sources of evaluation, can equally serve as methods of knowledge with respect to that particular value that represents truth. One thus forgets that truth only obtains its proper value by embodying within itself the necessary rules of verification, and one applies to it intuitive procedures, which have the specific character that they can only be used in the approach to noncognitive but lived values. In short, we give to the coordination of values an ontological status they cannot sustain, in order to legitimatize the illusory passage from evaluative intuitions to an impossible epistemological intuition. These are, however, the kind of sophisms denounced by Kant at least two centuries ago.[4]

Additional Note on Ontology and the "Inadequacies" of Science

The "philosopher" readily conceives of science in a positivist form and reduces it to a catalog of facts and laws. Scientific procedures are similarly only considered as techniques for the description of facts and the establishment of laws. This is why philosophy reserves for itself the right to discuss the *value* of science, and, hence, its *truth*.

It then criticizes science for not taking account of:

1. Man
2. Being, and also

[4] A nice example of this complete neglect of Kantianism in the rising generation is F. Brunner's book, *Science et realité* ("Philosophie de l'esprit," Aubier). One can summarize it as follows: 1. There is only a true science in God; 2. Science knows nothing of God; 3. Therefore it is "anthropomorphic," relative, imperfect, etc., while the notions of transcendent finality, etc., alone constitute valid knowledge because they are nonanthropocentric. It is regrettable that the divine wisdom, of which F. Brunner appears to be a familiar, has not given him more complete information about "science," from which he has remained at an uncomfortable distance in order to speak confidently of it and to offer us simply the substitution of Brunnerocentrism for anthropomorphism. One would have expected from such a theological mind a little more propriety in his accusations before declaring, for example, "that science in its naive naturalism cannot overcome . . . the exasperating opposition of subject and object" (pp. 149–50), as if he understood the manifold relationships which mathematics, physics, biology, and psychology admit of in this respect.

3. The meaning of facts.

These three criticisms often amount only to one: ontology (or rather the ontic) brings us back to a metaphysics of meaning, and there is only one meaning for man. But:

(a) Either the clarification of meaning arises from a critique of knowledge; in this case philosophy is indistinguishable from epistemology;

(b) Either it goes beyond epistemological inquiry, the meaning then being constituted or exhibited in *praxis* and in *history* (cf. *Critique de la raison dialectique*).

But what is it which makes history or *praxis* intelligible? An immediate intuition? This is an epistemological concept, which there is every reason for discussing as such. The "necessity of things"? But then, why philosophers? (unless it is in order to philosophize about engagement, but then it is engagement and not philosophy which elaborates meaning).

Let us then consider the three criticisms separately:

(1) *Science does not take account of man*

If man = self, unique and irreplaceable, we have nothing to say. But philosophy has little else to teach me than the revelation of my freedom, no matter how, on the other hand, I may be determined by my body, society, and history, which then leads to a philosophy of values, wisdom, or prolegomena to my wisdom.

Otherwise, man is the object of knowledge. The idea that man as object is the inessential phenomenal arises from a twofold sophism or twofold superstition for:

– nothing prevents the possibility of a psychology (or of an ethnology, etc.), of the subject as subject (except in the above sense, which forces us back into the ineffable);

– even metaphysics today seeks for the essence of man starting from phenomena, or, as we will see later on, from discourse about phenomena.

(2) *Science does not take account of Being*

Heidegger, *Introduction à la metaphysique*, French translation, 1958, P.U.F.: "Philosophy is always directed to the primary and ultimate foundations of being," but he adds: "and this in a fashion that man himself expressly finds there an interpretation and also an intuition of ends concerning man-as-being" (p. 17).

But we can then say:

(a) That an inquiry into Being finally ends at an inquiry into the *foundation* of values.[5]

(b) Heidegger's work, for example, constantly asserts the tragic divorce of Being and knowledge. But in accepting this divorce, one can infer either that knowledge abandons the absolute from the very fact that it sets itself the task of circumscribing these problems, or that the inquiries are directed differently. Knowledge describes in this latter case the outside layer or the realization of Being on the various levels that the method of knowledge is able to elaborate; philosophy itself is not a knowledge of Being: it tries to ensure its revelation. And from this fact it tends to mysticism or to poetry, and cannot escape this undoubtedly respectable calling. But the dialogue between the logos of knowledge and the logic of Hölderlin is broken. The divorce of Being and knowledge can also show the inadequacy of science to reveal Being (something it has never claimed to do), which marks the failure of metaphysics as productive of truths. This is why despite the severe criticism that Heidegger makes of the concept of value, it is on the plane of values that metaphysical reflection takes its impulse and inspiration.

(c) An indication of this is that a philosophy of this kind carries out its inquiries on the level of *speech*, and not on that of language insofar as language has become an object of scientific study. To philosophize is to translate. Heidegger's two lectures *Was heisst Denken?* are concerned one with translating an expression of Nietzsche, the other in translating two verses of Parmenides and to translate them *into Greek*. It is not that the word thinks: there is no longer a boundary between the lan-

---

[5] Heidegger criticizes Nietzsche (*op. cit.*, p. 213) for not having understood that the origin of the concept of value was a problem, and for not having thus "attained the central problem of philosophy."

guage of Being and its metalanguage. A strange conception of thought, which challenges fact and deduction, in order to remain content with its unaided practice. It will be said that Heidegger has never even attempted to give a critique of *science*, which is much to his credit: one can therefore assume that scientists speak meaningfully and to the point about the subject matter they have modestly restricted themselves to. But this is also to overlook that scientists question their own field of inquiry, that the being of microphysics is not the same as that of Galilean physics, that the mathematical being of today is no longer the same as that of Euclid and of Descartes, etc. Why not then begin ontology by this inquiry into the being of science (or of the sciences)?

(Let it not be said that this being is that of things: it is well and truly being—for—the subject, for the knowing subject, of course.)

(d) Finally, *Sein and Zeit* distinguishes the existential analysis of *beings* from the existential analysis that is ontological, in opposition to the ontic. But only the first part of the program is realized. Are we rash in assuming that this marks not the failure but the *impossibility* of metaphysics?

(3) *Science does not take account of the meaning of facts*

This criticism, which comes up again nowadays, can mean two things.

(a) In the first sense, it means that science only deals with contingent facts. We shall return to this conception, which is not even that of positivism. On the other hand, science has never limited itself to the "hunt of Pan." The co-ordination of facts and laws, the simulation of facts by models, the elaboration of theories are all equally procedures by which meaning is constituted. And there is no doubt that however "delimited" be the problems, this meaning is usually more profound than that obtained by direct intuition. It has sometimes been claimed that in passing from facts to theory the scientist passes from pure science to philosophy. And indeed, the scientist cannot on occasion escape the need to philosophize. But it is contrary to the nature of the scientific spirit to imagine that "theory" or "meaning" can be elaborated by means of a Reason different from the reason that gives rise to science. Of course, the methods—if method is to mean technique of approach, etc.—are not necessarily the same at each level of elaboration: but science does not sanction two sources of truth, two modes of judgment, and in this it differs from philosophy. Brunschvicg (*Écrits philosophiques*, Vol. III, *Sciences et religion*, P.U.F.) in this connection refers to Pascal's distinction, and shows excellently that the scientific spirit today is necessarily both *subtle* and *geometrical*.

(b) In a second sense, the criticism would be that science is only directed toward the objective, and methodically neglects subjective meanings—the psychology of behavior has been criticized for this. One looks for adrenalin or grimaces, but not for anger, etc. But there is a psychology of conduct (to which we will return): scientific linguistics does not limit itself to dictionary meanings, and the study of meaning is in no way the prerogative of reflective philosophy.

To sum up, philosophy would most certainly be in the right if it was concerned with fields of inquiry where science does not go, where it does not wish to go, cannot go for the moment. But there is no justification for its belief that these fields are its preserve *in aeternum*. And it is in no way able to prove that its problems are by nature different from those that scientific Reason proposes to attack. Science is only concerned with appearance? But according to a well-known formula, of all the paths which lead to Being, appearance is perhaps still the surest. As for marking the present limits of scientific knowledge, is this not a mark of scientific thought itself? No philosopher could make a list as long and as self-critical of the mistakes and inadequacies of science as could a scientist.

The Ambitions
of a Philosophical
Psychology

Chapter Four

THE PHRASE "philosophical psychology" can be taken in two
very different senses, only the second of which will concern us.
The first covers every form of psychology developed by thinkers
who were also philosophers. The phrase "philosophical psychology" as thus used has no intrinsic significance, for before the
emergence of a scientific psychology philosophers have either
been concerned with purely speculative inquiries, using psychological data as a starting point for metaphysical developments,
or with the beginnings of concrete psychology, the forerunner
of the future positive psychology, or with both at once. F. L.
Mueller in a recent book on *L'histoire de la psychologie de
l'Antiquité à nos jours*, some theses of which will be critically
examined in Chapter Five, has excellently portrayed the main
features of the psychology elaborated by the great philosophers,
with which we shall not be concerned here. But it is important
to avoid all ambiguity and to recall clearly (cf. also Chapter
Two under B) that, if scientific psychology only began in the
nineteenth century in an experimental form, it has over a long
period been prepared by more or less methodical or accidental
observations.

By "philosophical psychology" today one has rather in mind a
psychology that endeavors to be independent of scientific psychology and whose aim it is to complete or even supplant it. We are
solely concerned here with this intellectual trend, for it is neces-

sary to discuss its legitimacy and the validity of the results obtained respecting our general problem of the possibility of a philosophical knowledge distinct from scientific knowledge. And this general problem takes on here a specific form of particular interest from our point of view, since philosophical psychology is related to a delimited field, given as different from that of metaphysics and relative to the "phenomena" alone. This new philosophical psychology can in this respect be traced back to Maine de Biran, for even if in his time scientific psychology was unaware of its autonomy, and even if Biranian psychology was only critical of that of the empiricists, Biran believed in the Kantian distinction of noumena and phenomena and took care to limit his inquiry to the latter alone, which did not prevent him from extending it in the form of idealist speculations.

As philosophical psychology is nevertheless always an essential part of a major metaphysical system (otherwise it would quickly end in a positive inquiry, which is not the same as positivism), it is naturally subject to "variations" in some way congenital, which is its first distinctive mark. One might reply that this occurs just as much in the field of scientific psychology, which is certainly true if one takes up a static point of view. But the great difference is that experimental psychologists undertake cooperative research on the methods of verification that enable them to reach agreement. There is an "International Union of Scientific Psychology" grouping all the psychological societies of the world, except those of which there is no evidence of their effective work.[1] The Central Committee of the Union has for some years been made up of fifteen members from different psychological schools. Of these there are at the moment two representatives from Eastern Europe and two priests, without there being the least difficulty as to the drawing up of the programs of International Congresses or of cooperation in research projects: the latter ought, among other things to include comparative studies so as to verify the generality of certain facts and see

[1] This means that the association through these societies covers more than 40,000 members invited to International Congresses.

if they depend on the cultural milieux. I find it difficult to imagine an International Committee concerned with philosophical psychology that would exhibit the same harmony if it included within it Thomists, dialectical materialists, phenomenologists, Bergsonians, Kantians, rationalists, etc.

(A) A first problem is relative to the very subject matter of philosophical psychology. It is possible to achieve a verbal agreement if we say that it is derived from phenomena, but phenomenology interprets such a concept quite differently than does "scientific psychology"; and "rational psychology," still taught by Thomists, ignores on principle the distinction between phenomena and noumena, a distinction denied, moreover, by many other philosophers also or accepted in very different ways. This is not the question however, which is: (1) whether philosophical psychology is concerned with "facts" or with something else called "essences" or "intuitions"; (2) whether that which we designate by the terms "intention" or "meaning" derives from one or other of these possibilities; and (3) to establish whether the subject matter of philosophical psychology is relative to consciousness alone or not, and if the demarcation line between philosophical and scientific psychologies is to be drawn as a function of this consciousness or of introspection.

From the point of view of facts or of essences, the philosophical psychologies of Maine de Biran or of Bergson both claim that they deal with facts and will continue to do so, but believe that they are better able to arrive at the facts than is empiricism or laboratory psychology, and that they provide the best interpretations of them. It is therefore worthwhile discussing these philosophical psychologies on the field of facts.

On the other hand, the psychology of Sartre, etc., claims to transcend facts in favor of essences, but it is doubtful whether he has understood what a "fact" is in the field of psychology in view of his surprising definition of it: "To expect a *fact*, is by definition to expect the isolated, it is for positivism, to prefer the 'accident' to the essential, the contingent to the necessary, disorder to order; it is in principle to reject the essential in the future: This is left over for a later date when we will have collected sufficient facts. Psychologists do not take into account that it is just as impossible to attain the essence by the accumulation of contingent fact than to arrive at unity by indefinitely adding numbers to the right of 0.99. If their only aim is to accumulate knowledge of factual detail, we have nothing to say; except that we do not see the interest of these fact-collecting studies. But if in their modesty they are moved by the hope, laudable in itself, that one will later bring about on the basis of their monographs an anthropological synthesis, they plainly contradict themselves." [2]

In psychological circles ("psychology attracts psychopaths," Claparède said) one can certainly come across persons having the mentality of butterfly or postcard collectors, as sometimes happens in philosophical circles where one finds schizoids attaining "essences" much too easily. But to describe laboratory work in the way Sartre has done, definitely shows that he has not worked in one and that he has not the least idea what an experimental inquiry is.

A "fact" as conceived by scientists exhibits three characteristics of which we may ask whether the first and the third do not approximate to that which Sartre calls the "essence," the second serving as a control of the two others. Each scientific "fact" is: (a) an answer to a question; (b) a verification or a "reading off"; (c) a sequence of interpretations, already implicit in the very manner of asking the question, as well (unfortunately or fortunately) as in the verification as such, or the "reading off" of experience, and explicit in the manner of understanding the answer given by reality to the question asked.

(a) A fact is first an answer to a question. If Sartre had consulted psychologists before judging them in the light of his own genius, he would have learned that they do not wait on the accident but begin by setting themselves problems. These problems are not equally fruitful, but still they are problems: for

[2] *Esquisse d'une théorie des émotions*, 2nd ed., 1948, p. 5 (quoted by F. L. Mueller, *loc. cit.*, p. 406).

example, to see whether in the developing subject, i.e. the child, integers are directly constructed starting from class logic by biunivocal correspondence and the construction of a "class of equivalent classes" as Frege and B. Russell thought, or whether the construction is more complex and presupposes the concept of order. I do not know if this problem has anything to do with "essences," because I have never really understood what an essence is, and I have found among philosophers answers that varied a little too much. I know, however, that Frege believed he had found the essence of number in biunivocal and reciprocal correspondence, independently of all psychologism, and that Frege's writings led Husserl to look for "essences" in place of "contingent facts." I therefore believe that a well-formulated problem is always conceptual and has to a lesser or greater extent some of the characteristics of that which some philosophers call essences; and that the problem selected here as an example comes pretty close to the "essence" of number, with roughly this important difference (to which we will return), that instead of looking for the essence in myself, despite the favorable preconceptions I harbor in this respect, I believe it prudent to study it among children who have not been subjected to the sophistications of theory or have remained unaffected by them. It is true that a fact can sometimes appear to resemble an "accident," as in the case of the apple that fell near Newton, but the accident only became a "fact" because Newton asked certain questions. If Adam had let fall the apple that Eve offered him he would perhaps have escaped original sin, and we with him, but he would not as such have discovered gravitation.

(b) A fact then involves a verification, or a "reading off" of experience, and it is here that the most serious misunderstandings arise from the point of view of essence and accident, because philosophers have at will simplified or obscured problems (and obscured because simplified), whether they have been empiricists, positivists, or phenomenologists, etc., instead of using the only possible procedure that will enable them to obtain a clear view of the matter: to study experimentally subjects in the process of verifying a fact, so as to analyze what this verification consists in. This analysis is far from having been taken as far as it should, but we have begun this at the *Centre d'épistémologie génétique* and now have enough evidence [3] to be able to assert that the experimental study of verification contradicts the interpretation given to it by empiricism (or, as F. Gonseth said of our studies: "The empirical study of experience refutes empiricism"), and with it the interpretation of those who in order to criticize "fact" conceive it in the empiricist manner.

As Duhem has shown a long time ago in the field of physical facts, a verification is always bound up with a system of interpretation or, as he said, with a "theory." What is surprising is that this is the same at all levels. A child shown a series of vertical rods ordered at equal distances apart (the tops forming in this case an inclined straight line) or decreasing in distance (the line being in this case hyperbolic), and asked to compare two perceived distances at the beginning and toward the end of the series, treats them quite differently according to whether or not he has grasped the idea of the tops forming a line. He perceives a line as horizontal or oblique according to whether or not he has the "idea" of looking for points of reference external to the figure. From the perceptual level onward, the verification of fact is therefore bound up with an interpretative structuring. This is even more so as soon as it is a question of complex verifications, as in the case of the formation of number and of biunivocal correspondence [quoted under (a)]. I believe I have "verified" the existence of a level where the child does not believe in the conservation of number (therefore in the permanence of equivalence by correspondence) as soon as one changes the spatial arrangement of the elements: but has my verification been sufficiently "objective" so that other observers can "verify" the same "facts"? Many of my readers have had the same doubts, and I have only been reassured in reading the results of control experiments made in other countries.

[3] See *Études d'épistémologie génétique*, Presses Universitaires de France, Vols. V–X.

Even verification is conceptualized, and the "reading off" of experience is never a simple "reading off" and involves in reality a complete structuring. We are a long way from the "accident" or from the "disorder" Sartre speaks of, and even if it is true that the grasping of the object involves a succession of approximations comparable to the passage from 0.99 to 1 (and I challenge Sartre to attain the limit 1 better than we can, although he has the comfortable impression of directly getting there by "intuition"), it is this succession of approximations that one refers to as the achieving of objectivity, starting from the inevitable subjective errors. To describe this procedure by the expression "accumulation of contingent fact" merely shows that he knows nothing whatever about that intellectual stringency which objectivity involves, and we may then ask whether this is not the distinctive mark of philosophical psychology.

(c) A "fact" therefore presupposes implicit interpretations resulting from the status of the problem and from its verification, but it is only a scientific fact if it leads, on the other hand, to an explicit interpretation that ensures its understanding. Such an understanding may be prudently deferred ("we leave this for later"), this will certainly happen, and we have here a new mark of objectivity. But this does not at all prevent a provisional or hypothetical interpretation, and if this was not done we would not try to collect other facts.

The condemnation of "facts" whose value we have tried to estimate does not at all raise the problem of essence and accident, but is rather evidence of a difficulty in understanding the scope of objectivity. We need therefore to examine the validity of a direct psychological knowledge of "essences" and particularly to ask if a "subjective" knowledge is possible; in other words if, because psychology is knowledge of the subject and his subjectivity, one can from this very fact be justified in speaking of knowledge in treating subjectively and not objectively this subjectivity inherent in the subject. The main reason why phenomenological psychology is opposed to the facts is plainly that it believes that knowledge dehumanizes itself in neglecting its existential roots, because the foundations of psychism are irrational: emotion is a magical attitude, the image of an absence of the object, which tries to pass itself off as being present, etc. This thesis would mean not only that intelligence is not the whole of mental life, which is evident, but also that the rational structures are only very secondary superstructures, instead of being related to the structures of the organism and to those of the general coordination of actions, as I would assume myself. As these general questions cannot in the present state of knowledge give rise to any demonstrated solution, the irrationalist hypotheses remain plausible and this is not therefore the question for the moment. The problem is whether in order to understand the irrational we need to make use of an irrational mode of thought, or if the latter runs the risk of simply becoming a fictional description as opposed to intelligence, which (even if it is only an unimportant superstructure for the subject and does not hold for the deeper structures of his being) can, among other things, understand even disorder. For example, in order to understand randomness, which is our model of the irrational, neither the physicist nor the mathematician finds it necessary to think "at random." That in order to understand their patients some psychiatrists may find it necessary to enter into their skin, to think irrationally, and to adopt toward the patient an existential and not a theoretical attitude, is perfectly legitimate and explains the success of phenomenology among some contemporary psychiatrists; however, it is only an essentially practical point of view whose success proves nothing scientifically. But when a philosophical psychologist claims to grasp the irrational by taking on its form, this raises more difficulties, for this experience then requires to be conceptualized and every conceptualization is a return to the rational.

Therefore, not wishing to conform to the demands of scientific objectivity, which increasingly aspires (see B) to understand all mental life including subjectivity in each of its aspects, even irrational, and being unable to escape the need for conceptualization, the phenomenological psychologists have tried to elaborate concepts that express conscious activities better than do "positive" concepts: such are the fundamental notions of *intention* and *meaning*. The question we have to look into is whether these are valid notions (taken in their general sense and independently of the particular applications that have been made of them to the problems of emotion, imagery, or perception) and whether, being valid, they are really alien to the conceptualization of scientific psychology.

The notion of intention comprises two meanings, of which the second extends the first on an epistemological level. From the psychological point of view, it is the assertion that every conscious state expresses an activity "directed toward" (let us not say a goal, for this is already an interpretation) an end state sought after and desired. All mental life would therefore involve intentionality, and in failing to understand the latter we would impoverish its essential dimension. From the epistemological point of view, Husserl's "intention" derives from the *intentio*, which his teacher Brentano retained from Thomism after having left the Church: it is still intentionality but which, on the conceptual level, can attain the forms or essences when, in knowledge, the subject "becomes" the object not materially but intentionally.

Intentionality is in fact a fundamental dimension of mental life, account of which has been taken in varying degrees since psychology has abandoned the sort of mechanistic atomism that associationism had proposed as the only model. The actual term "intention" is perhaps less used than others, but the idea is general. But it is above all with regard to this notion that Dilthey, Spranger, Jaspers, etc., have developed the well-known opposition between "understanding" and "explaining": understanding shows itself intuitively in the intention of others, while explanation refers to the causal mechanism. It is this opposition, which has become classical in the German-speaking world, which has in some quarters increased the anti-experimental tendencies. It is clear that phenomenological psychology in speaking of "intentions" is concerned with the field of "understanding" and believes from this very fact that it counters the "explanatory" and objective attitudes of scientific psychology.

But if the distinction between explanation and understanding is well-founded, as corresponding to the two different points of view of the subject's consciousness and of behavior considered in its completeness, it is futile to see in this a logical antithesis, for we have here the model of two complementary and not antithetical points of view, and even complementary in the usual and logical sense of the term and not in the physical sense (where the complementaries are alternatives and cannot occur simultaneously). It follows that, even when one does not speak explicitly of intentionality in a theory of an "explanatory" type, the notion can play a central role, but in another terminology.

If I can quote myself as an example, all the data I have tried to analyze in terms of a sensori-motor schematism and of assimilatory schemes have an intentional character. It is because of this that the phenomenological philosopher Aron Gurwitsch of New York, much more in touch with psychology than his French-speaking colleagues, uses my concept of assimilation to justify his arguments. Even before language begins, the young infant reacts to objects not by a mechanical set of stimulus-response associations but by an integrative assimilation to schemes of action, which impress a direction on his activities and include the satisfaction of a need or an interest. Although at first unrelated to each other as a function of the various as yet uncoordinated possibilities inherent in the body itself, these schemes become coordinated as a result of reciprocal assimilation, and one can speak of the strict intentionality of these coordinations.[4] In no way intellectualist, since the scheme of assimilation is at one and the same time motivation and understanding, this mode of interpretation is being applied by S. Escalona to the affective reactions of the first year, and we know their importance in later life.

[4] And of an intentionality that is creative of meanings, *i.e.* of the kind of realities the phenomenologists describe in terms of "essences" when they rightly see in intentionality the indissociable bond between subject and object.

In thus substituting assimilation for the mechanical concept of association (and this naturally holds a *fortiori* for the rest of development), intentionality is incorporated into an "explanatory" point of view, since the assimilatory mechanism is an extension of biological mechanisms, without at all excluding the point of view of subjective "understanding." In particular, in place of finality, a subjective concept entirely relative to the subject's consciousness itself, a parallelism is introduced between this egocentric notion, which would be illusory from the explanatory point of view, and a causal system changing from a state of disequilibrium to one of equilibrium, the equilibrium being itself explained by regulations involving loops or self-regulations.

As for the notion of meaning, which some philosophers go so far as to make the criterion of philosophical psychology in opposition to scientific psychology, the latter, on the contrary, gives an increasingly important role to it, in complete agreement with Saussurian linguistics and Levi-Strauss's cultural anthropology. In the perspective just noted, the sensori-motor schematism is already imbued with meaning well before language and representation, since to assimilate an object to such schemes is to confer meaning on it. But the meanings at this level are as yet only signs or perceptual signals. With the semiotic function there appears, on the other hand, differentiated meanings: linguistic signs and the symbols specific to symbolic play, to mental images, etc. Sartre's formula, according to which the image is an absence of being trying to pass itself off as something present, is only a fictional description of all representation, in which a differentiated meaning, whether it be symbol or sign, enables an absent reality to be recalled. "Magical act," says Sartre, "incantation intended to make the object thought about appear"; admittedly, but the verb is also magic, the algebraic sign is just as much magic, the only difference being that the image evokes perceptual data (without deriving it as such from perception), while the sign evokes conceptual realities. Certainly there is magic if one begins by deciding not to "explain" anything so as to limit oneself to understanding intuitively, but it can then be asked if the magic is inherent in Sartre, whose mode of knowledge recalls here the *co-naissance* of Claudel, or if it is in the subject. For someone concerned to observe the subject without trying to ascribe magic to him at least on these points, the appearance of the symbol in image form about one and a half to two years of age extends imitation; for imitation is a kind of representation worked out in concrete acts, which once sufficient virtuosity has been achieved is freed from its initial motor context to function in varied forms, *i.e.* without the first imitative copy being made in the presence of the model, and finally is internalized, just like language when it becomes internal speech. The mental image then owes its formation to an internalized imitation whose powers are as yet very limited in the young child (despite the imagination ascribed to him), and requires to be completed by imitative symbolic play as yet external but then becoming increasingly developed under the influence of thought.

In short, neither intentionality deeply rooted in mental life nor the absolutely general role of the notion of meaning, which could well be the most important cognitive characteristic of consciousness as compared with the dynamic aspect characteristic of intentions, is the preserve of philosophical psychology: these are also notions occurring in contemporary psychology.

(B) Will we therefore find in the notions of consciousness and introspection criteria for the subject matter of philosophical psychology? Although we come near it, it is just on this point that misunderstandings, involuntary or sometimes almost deliberate, are the most tenacious and have the weightiest consequences. In his *Psychologie Contemporaine*, intended like his *Histoire de la Psychologie* to rehabilitate philosophical psychology, F. L. Mueller makes, for example, the surprising remark with regard to the present tendency to consider the animal as a *subject* and not as an *automaton:* "Can one deny that this recognition of the animal as *subject* opens up a 'set of problems' of a philosophical order? One could say that here again the philosophy expelled by the door returns by the window" (p. 81).[5] Let us not take too seriously the term "the philosophy," which has the absurd consequence of excluding from "the philosophy" that of Descartes, who believed in animal-machines. But what is surprising is not that philosophy interests itself in the subject, since everything, including the organism, can give rise to a set of philosophical problems (cf. the fine work of F. Meyer and the metaphysical studies of Ruyer), but that according to Mueller the subject does not seem to be the concern of scientific psychology and that its mere introduction makes philosophy return by the window. For more than forty years now I have constantly been stressing the "activities of the subject" in the case of the sensorimotor mechanisms and of perception as well as in that of the "reading off" of experience and intelligence at all these levels; I did not know that I lived with such badly closed windows.

Let us therefore be clear and concise. If Watson and Soviet reflexology have wanted to or appeared to banish consciousness from their field of studies, Watson's lineal descendants (adherents of so-called behavior theory) speak constantly today of conscious activities and Russian psychologists continue to be interested in the problem of consciousness. The most widely held point of view in scientific psychology today is that which Janet, Claparède, Pieron, and many others have called the "psychology of conduct," "conduct" being defined as behavior that includes consciousness.

And the proof that the adherents of the "psychology of conduct" do not neglect consciousness is that they look for its laws. Claparède has shrewdly noted that children of a certain age who

[5] This passage refers, among others, to F. J. J. Buytendijk, formerly professor at the Calvinist University of Amsterdam, then at the Catholic University of Utrecht, where he became converted to phenomenology after a brilliant career as an experimentalist. The author praises him for treating the animal as a subject when he had ceased to be productive in the field of animal psychology, but Mueller has not realized that the "objectivist" school of Lorenz and Tinbergen does this too and has similarly brought to light the spontaneous activities of the organism, but without ceasing to continue the search for causal connections (among others, by means of cybernetic models).

overgeneralize without taking differences into account, have much more difficulty when they are asked to compare two objects (a bee and a fly, etc.) to indicate their similarities rather than their differences. From which he has derived his "law of conscious realization" according to which consciousness is at first connected with an environmental situation blocking some activity, therefore with the reasons for this maladaptation and not with the activity itself, which does not give rise to reflection as long as it remains adapted. Consciousness thus proceeds from the periphery to the center and not inversely. It is true that Sartre disputes this (without proof) and does not believe in the unconscious. He is certainly right in attacking the authenticity of the unconscious nature of the Freudian "disguises," and I argued myself at the same time that the disguise due to the censor is never unconscious except with the subject's connivance.[6] But Sartre forgets—and we shall try to see why—the unconscious character of processes that have never been conscious, of which we only become conscious with difficulty and by a retrospective effort of reflection. We are thus only conscious of the results of our thought and not of its mechanisms (whence Binet's witticism, "Thought is an unconscious activity of the mind"), except by a reflection liable to error and always incomplete.

Independently of the questions of conscious realization and of degrees of unconsciousness, it could be argued that scientific psychology nevertheless tends to neglect consciousness, given its general tendency to relate mental processes to organic processes. This is certainly true if we only consider its historical beginnings and the preliminary phases of research. But what is then completely overlooked and which is not at all to be seen in the philosophico-historic panoramas of Mueller, is the increasingly modern tendency to employ "abstract models" in all fields of psychology relative to cognitive functions like perception and

[6] See *La formation du symbole.* Delachaux & Niestlé (English translation, *Plays, Dreams and Imitation in Childhood,* Norton, 1951).

intelligence (but not exclusively: see the applications of information theory and the theory of games in Berlyne's studies on curiosity and interest, or the relations between decision theory and free-will). Let us first note that this is true even in psychophysiology and in neurology. Fessard has given a probability model of conditioning in the form of a differentiated stochastic network, and contemporary mechanico physiology looks to cybernetics and electronic computing devices (Ashby's homeostat, Turing machines, etc.) for its models. As far as intelligence is concerned, I have since my first studies in 1921 used logistic models, then probabilistic ones, and there are many other such models (theory of graphs, for instance). This increasingly general use of "abstract models" has in no way led to that mechanical picture of behavior and epiphenomenal consciousness that many associationist psychologists dreamed of at a time when, like the philosophers, they were satisfied with a simple reflection on facts that had already been collected methodically, although without being able as yet to use precise deductive methods. The use of these methods and mechanical models gives rise sooner or later to the idea that there is a structural isomorphism between the organization of the physical mechanism assumed to simulate the brain, and the organization of conscious thought (we will come back to this mechanism in connection with Bergson). There exists, however, a fundamental difference between them: while the machine operates causally in such a way that, for example, the mechanical equivalents of the numbers 2 and 3 when combined give the mechanical equivalent of 5 resulting from the nature of the circuits, transmission of energy, etc., dependent upon physical causality alone; conscious thought, on the other hand, deals with "pure meanings." The relations between the latter are not of a causal order but consist in "implications" in the wider sense, for $2 + 3$ is not the cause of 5 but the logical equivalent of 5, which it implies. And it is not because I now wish to answer phenomenological psychology that I thus oppose causality to the system of meanings and their implications, as I have defended this idea continuously since 1950 [7] and well before that I tried to show that the concept of assimilation substituted for that of association entails the concepts of meaning and implications between meanings. And Claparède already stated that for Pavlov's dog, in considering the dog as a subject (this for F. L. Mueller's information), the sound of the bell "implies" food, without which he would not salivate.

Scientific psychology cannot therefore be thought of as necessarily neglecting consciousness, and similarly it cannot be prevented from studying the "subject" (we have seen this in Chapter Three under D), and it is useless returning to this. On the other hand, the problem of introspection remains, and it is here that we come near to the essential difference between scientific and philosophical psychologies. But this difference is in no way connected, as might be believed, with the use of introspection as such. Certainly as a procedure it has its dangers and is fertile in systematic errors; this has been stressed by all. But combined with the study of conduct, introspection gives three sorts of data that are indispensable without, of course, speaking of lived experience, without which conduct would be meaningless. In the first place, the study of the subject's conscious realization in relation to his actual conduct is in general of great interest: for example, in the child the comparison between his conscious realization of the meaning of a term and the use he effectively makes of it. In the second place, the systematic errors of introspection are in themselves very significant. In the third place, the methods of controlled introspection systematically used by Binet and the Würzburg school, without giving them what they hoped for have, nevertheless, had decisive importance in showing the falsity of the associationist explanation of judgment and the secondary role of the image, conceived before verifications as an element of thought.

If this is the case, why is there a basic disagreement between

[7] See also *Traité de psychologie expérimentale*, by P. Fraisse and J. Piaget, Vol. I, Chapter III: "L'explication en psychologie."

the experimentalists and all those who, since V. Cousin "tortured his consciousness" in order to derive from its solemn platitudes, have dedicated themselves to an introspective psychology? The latter have ended up with doctrines which, although having at least the merit of abandoning common sense, are of such diversity that discussion with the experimentalist becomes impossible.

We see straightaway that there is definitely only one criterion distinguishing philosophical from scientific psychology: that is, when the philosopher speaks of consciousness, of the body itself (and he increasingly speaks of it), of "being in the world," of "being for others," or "in presence of the object," etc., he only relies on his own introspection without any attempt at verification, except in himself and on himself. Husserl tells us that an essential dimension of his psychology is that of the "intersubjective," but it still concerns an intersubjective if not lived by itself at least interpreted by itself and without "objective" verification. To talk to a philosopher about "objective" verification is to make him immediately believe that we intend to distort the "subject." All we ask of him, however, is not to treat his reader as the reader of a novel who judges its psychology according to whether or not he sympathizes with the author's characters, but as a simple and honest intellectual who wishes to believe you but would like to be given the means to do so.

Let us take an example from the field of pure introspection. It concerns some research recently carried out by A. Rey on an old suggestion of Claparède, who had asked him if he could make a correct motor image of his own body in rotation. Rey had replied that he believed he could, but years afterward an observation seemed to show that this image is very limited. This careful and repeated introspection did not satisfy him, however, and he then tried to test it by means of a detailed questionnaire made up of precise but not leading questions, and involving selection from succinctly worded alternatives. The answers given by a certain number of adults trained in psychological observation turned out to be very close to each other, which therefore gave an objective test of a simple introspective datum.[8]

What, we may ask with trepidation, would become of such an observation in Sartre's terminology if he made it on himself (carefully or by means of the pifometer)? However correct may be his "ontological" dialectic of his own body at first lived, then perceived by others (at the same time as those of others are known), then known as an object through the point of view of others (which does not seem so different from what J. M. Baldwin said long ago concerning the simultaneous genetic construction of the ego and the *alter* at the level of the first two years), Sartre's introspection is from the first directed by two philosophical postulates expressing his innermost self: the ontological and irrationalist postulates. This is very interesting for history but insufficient for truth, and has nothing to do with his reader's introspection when this reader has a different philosophy or is trying to come to terms with reality by correcting his philosophy in the light of it.

The ontological postulate is only of relative importance, for in most cases it only adds to the given data a verbal label or a declaration of principle. Sartre believes that he is able to attain being directly by means of intuition. Bergson believed this too, but according to Sartre he deceived himself. Some future philosophical fashion will attain "being" in another manner, and will show that Sartre in his turn has been seriously mistaken. This has little consequence, since as Kant has shown one hundred real thalers (or as one says today, having an ontological existence) only differs from the concept of a hundred thalers by a property that leaves the other qualities of the thalers unchanged. It is thus a matter of temperament if you like, to have the impression for each intuitive representation, of grasping being itself or of seeking to attain it by successive approximations (as in the passage of 0.99 to 1!). In order to understand how Sartre's realism applies to these free decisions that engage "all consciousness" and which will be imposed throughout life on every introspec-

[8] See *Archives de psychologie*, Vol. XXXVIII, pp. 256–74.

tion, one needs to read in the very interesting memoirs of Simone de Beauvoir her account of the time when Sartre, with a glass of beer in front of him, shouted with delight that thanks to Husserl we can at last give to this glass an ontological value. For myself, when I know my body through the vision of others, I prefer to speak of the coordination of points of view and to see in this one of the numerous stages of those general coordinations of actions and of points of view that constitute rationality, but it seems to me that adding the label "ontological" changes nothing at all in most questions.

On the other hand, we have much greater misgivings about the second postulate, that of irrationality, because it is of a kind to falsify all introspection, and if it is said that it is itself derived from introspection, we can ask whether this is peculiar to Jean-Paul Sartre's "self" or whether it is general. For Sartre "psychical causality," which is how he describes the relationships between meanings, is essentially irrational and "magical" and the psychologist who does not put himself within these "irrational connections" and does not take them as the "first datum of the psychical world" is only an intellectualist distorting reality. The reasons given for this magical irrationality, moreover, are so very odd and so bad as to make it quite apparent that it is a question of "rationalization," as the psychoanalysts put it, that is to say, once again, that it is necessary to look for their origin in the "decisions of the whole being" and not in pure observation. The reasons appealed to are in general "magical actions at a distance," as in situations where one sees oneself as known by others, or where the image renders "presence of the object" an "absence of the object," etc. But the characteristic of representative intelligence is to enable us to think of objects and events outside the perceptual field, and to call the fundamental act of rational knowledge magical is the height of an ontological anti-intellectualism. What would Sartre have said if instead of being concerned with his self he interested himself in the epistemology of a present-day astronomer computing the precise moment of an eclipse at the time of Julius Caesar or in the year 2722 after

Christ? He would have seen in this logico-mathematical deduction an overwhelming example of action at a distance and of "absence of being" becoming "presence of being," while regretting that this magic is disembodied in an abstract computation. If every act of intelligence is called irrational we then merely need to agree about terminology. For even in the case of P. Janet's patient who Sartre tells us became hysterical "in order" to attract magically the sympathy of her doctor, this magic interpreted at the same time as "intentionality" is not completely lacking in intelligence. But we still need to understand this obsession with irrationality in such an intelligent author; similarly, it has been shown that Bergson's "intuition" of trans-intellectual intention presupposes an elaboration and subtlety that are intelligent in the true sense of the word.

We merely need to refer to Sartre's dramatic work, which is much to be admired and which has in addition been completed by a philosophy that enables us better to see its human bearing on the coordination of values, even if from the epistemological point of view it appears as a projection of the self and of the social group in the representation of the universe. This work exhibits a surprising conviction in the irrationality of reality and, without needing to venture on a speculative psychoanalysis based on certain data given by Simone de Beauvoir, we can only try to understand why Sartre regards it as his duty and contribution to truth to proclaim the existence of irrationalities and to denounce the optimism of idealists or of intellectualists. But if we have here a valuable personal testimony due to a great personality, we must not confuse a lived experience with general psychological truths, and it is this confusion that characterizes the introspective method of philosophical psychology—not simply because it is introspective, but because it carries the fear of "objectivism" so far that it neglects "objectivity"—and the cult of subjectivity to the extent of fixing it on a particular self.

We may conclude from points (A) and (B) that the difference between scientific and philosophical psychologies is not due to the former being concerned with "facts" and the latter with "essences." For if one has understood what a scientific fact is (which, as we have seen, is not given to everyone), *i.e.* the verified answer to a problem, the intuition of essences could become a fact if we were given methods of verification. The difference is neither due to the concepts of intentionality or meaning, for these notions correspond to facts and are in ordinary use. The difference is not even due to the use of introspection, for if its use is restricted in scientific psychologies and it is used exclusively in philosophical psychologies, this would be merely a difference of degree. The only systematic difference that we have noted up to now is a difference of method. The scientific psychologist, even when he introspects, is interested in verification, which is not objectivism but *objectivity*, since one is concerned with consciousness. The philosophical psychologist under the pretext that he is concerned with intuitions, essences, intentions, and meaning, neglects all objectivity and verification as if they were intrinsic. His ideas are certainly full of interest, for every newly formulated problem is of interest, but they cannot be assimilated as long as there is no attempt to give or even look for criteria of verification. When late in life the psychologist Buytendijk, who had carried out excellent studies in animal psychology, became converted to phenomenology, he published among other things studies on the psychology of women and on football, which have somewhat saddened his friends but which seemed not to be based on introspection, since he is neither an Amazon nor a European champion. Despite their penetrating character, as is the case with everything he does, these studies differ essentially from his earlier work by a somewhat disturbing form of impressionism, as if phenomenological psychology, even when concerned with phenomena external to the self, consisted in describing them as refracted by the latter.

It is therefore on this essential point that we differ. All valid knowledge presupposes a decentration. The whole of the history of science is made up of decentrations, from the so-called primitive peoples who believed they could order the stars by their seasonal feasts, or from Aristotle's geocentricism to Newton, who still, however, believed in the absolute value of his measuring rods and his clocks, and down to Einstein, who has rid us of these last centrations—last until the next decentrations occur. Genetic psychology observes an analogous process in the development of individual perception and intelligence. I am well aware that Merleau-Ponty has said of my theory of decentration that it puts itself at the point of view of God himself. He exaggerates somewhat, but it is nonetheless sad to see men as able as the phenomenological psychologists devalue their ideas in subordinating them to a method that brings us back to new centrations, all the more tyrannical, since they are excused on philosophical grounds.

(C) If poor Maine de Biran had been able to guess where his method would lead to in the century of existentialism, he would have confined himself to physiological psychology. But he believed in introspection, and it is now necessary to do a little history in order to see whether this exclusive use of introspection has led the great philosophers of the past to the same errors of centration on the self as the phenomenological psychologists, even among men of a modesty as charming as was that of Maine de Biran. At the contrary risk of immodesty, I will add that Biranian thought interests me more as an individual, for in his fine book on *La perception de la causalité* A. Michotte regards my ideas on the sensori-motor origins of causality as a renewal of the famous thesis of Maine de Biran. It will therefore be useful for our purpose to compare a doctrine based on introspective data with an interpretation drawn from the first two years of life.

But before coming to causality, let us first recall the well-known error, due to introspection, which Maine de Biran has committed in connection with the feeling of effort, and which has falsified the rest of the doctrine on those questions where effort enters in. Maine de Biran, who appreciated Leibniz's reintroduction of the notions of finality and force, took up again the Cartesian *Cogito* in the light of these two concepts. And as introspection is always, in any case, a structuring of the so-called immediate data and not their direct intuition, this structuring

L

is naturally influenced by the ideas of the knowing subject who observes his individual self (we have just seen this clearly enough for Sartre). Therefore, introspecting the *cogito* in his self, Biran discovered that it is essentially force and finality and found the synthesis of these two properties in the consciousness of voluntary effort conceived as originating in a direct and centrifugal manner from the self, as it appears to introspection. We have here one of the clearest examples of introspective illusion when consciousness remains divorced from the rest of conduct.

From the first, W. James in a famous article that appeared in *Mind* around 1880, has shown that there is no sensation of innervation, and that consequently in muscular effort we do not experience the transmission of the efferent or centrifugal neural impulses. The process is therefore centripetal and we become conscious of effort as soon as we meet resistance. But P. Janet has shown that the experience of effort is one of those elementary experiences whose distinctive character corresponds to a "regulation" of action, i.e. to an activation or to a termination of an act. It is therefore the conduct connected with the effort that needs to be analyzed if we wish to understand the experience which expresses this regulative conduct. Following J. M. Baldwin and J. Philippe, Janet then verified that effort is a regulation of positive activation, as fatigue is a regulation of negative activation and joy and sadness are the regulations of termination according to success or failure. It depends essentially on an acceleration, that is to say on a reinforcement of the energies necessitated by the action: a cyclist proceeding at his normal pace makes no effort, but he does if he accelerates, if he proceeds at a faster pace than usual, or if he fights against increasing fatigue. As a regulation of acceleration or reinforcement, effort is no longer an energetic emanation from the "self" in Maine de Biran's sense. The self is not a "force," since the energies involved are organic, but a regulator which controls its output: or rather it is the system of meanings, values, intentions, etc., which translate in terms of consciousness the regulations of the whole action of which the self is the expression.

We thus see that it is a far cry from the introspective data to the real dynamics of conduct. Ordinary global introspection is not mistaken when it sees in the self the origin of effort, but it is correct only to the extent in which it does not analyze and limits itself to serving the ends of action. By transferring this utilitarian function into a cognitive method, introspective psychology runs the risk of overlooking the mechanisms whose intimate knowledge is useless for action, and which only a psychology of conduct can isolate in giving introspective data their true status, which is not cognitive.

This initial inadequacy of analysis then explains the difficulties inherent in the Biranian theory of causality. Hume believed he had eliminated this concept by reducing it purely to habitual succession without any objective connection of apparent necessity, and resulting simply from the coercive force of subjective associations and habits. Maine de Biran had the great merit, on the other hand, of looking for the origin of the idea of causality not in an external succession of any kind whatsoever, but in action itself where we can order the succession of acts by means of our intentions, and where consequently there occurs between the antecedents and the consequences a connection irreducible to simple association and justifying the notion of causality as a productive act. But what is the nature of such a connection, whose psychological analysis is extraordinarily complex because of the interference of physiological factors and consciousness (we will shortly return to this with respect to the principle of parallelism criticized by Bergson) and whose epistemological analysis can lead one into two opposite paths? One of these is the critical or Kantian interpretation, which Biran knew well since his own analyses were on the level of phenomena and not of noumena. The phenomenal data of the internal world are interpreted by the knowing subject as are those of the external world, that is to say the subject introduces by means of his understanding a rational connection between the antecedents and the consequents. The necessity peculiar to causality thus results from an *a-priori* relationship for Kant, or simply deductive as for Descartes (*causa seu ratio*), but always a relationship due to intelligence in its structuring of the given. The other path which Maine de Biran followed is, on the contrary, pre-critical (he wanted it to be transcritical) or intuitionist. It consists in looking for the causal connection in the phenomenon itself, with the hope that if the phenomena in general give the simple regular succession in which Hume believed, the internal phenomena connected with action itself will give a direct intuition or immediate apperception (a) of the cause; (b) of the effect; and above all (c) of the experienced and lived passage between cause and effect.

In limiting himself to his inadequate analysis of effort, Maine de Biran discovers these three terms: the cause is the self, origin of voluntary and muscular effort, the effect is an external modification of the self since it expresses itself at first by a resistance which denotes the externality of the object on which we act, and the experienced passage from the cause to the effect is directly given by the synchronism between voluntary and muscular effort: by "the absolute simultaneity of will and movement." [9]

[9] And "explain as one may how the cerebral impulses activate the nerves and by them the muscles, one will no better understand . . . the efficacity of the will in voluntary movement," *Oeuvres*, Vol. XI, p. 415 (quoted by D. Voutsinas, *La psychologie de Maine de Biran*, p. 95). This passage then admits: (1) a stream of nervous impulses proceeding from the brain to the periphery; (2) the fact that it corresponds to the primitive fact of synchronism between "will and movement"; and (3) the assumption that an explanation divorced from this centrifugal stream of impulses will not weaken the evidence for the causal character of this force inherent in the self which is voluntary effort. Without saying explicitly that we are conscious of the centrifugal stream of nervous impulses, for Maine de Biran did not wish to cross "the gap which separates the field of psychology from that of physiology," the above passage implies this consciousness; and the proof lies in Maine de Biran's refusal to accept Destutt de Tracy's distinction between the willed movement and the experienced movement during the movement of our limbs: "You abstract . . . the relative experience of effort from that of the force inherent in the self which originated it, which only knows itself in itself and by itself . . . ; as soon as one presupposes an experienced movement, it is also necessary to admit the conditions and the specific character under which alone it can be experienced . . ." (Quoted by Voutsinas, *op. cit.*, p. 268).

The Biranian interpretation of causality, being based on the purely psychologically given, admits, as does that of Hume, of direct experimental verification, not by introspection, since it is both judge and party and we have seen its errors with regard to the feeling of effort, but by a study of the actual origin of causality at the ages where it originates, *i.e.* from the first year. We will therefore give a general summary of the main results of such verification during the sensori-motor period (0 to 18–24 months), then from the period of the formation of operations (2 to 7–8 and from 7 to 11–12 years).

At the sensori-motor level, which is basic for our present discussion, causality begins from three to four months from the point of view of the subject. For example, the infant discovers by chance that by pulling a cord which hangs from the roof of his cot he can shake, rock and rattle the celluloid toys (which contain small shot) attached to the roof. The proof that he sees causality in this is that later on, the roof being cleared of toys, a new object has merely to be hung up there when he immediately reaches for the cord and pulls on it looking expectantly at the object. This causality is straight away so strongly held and generalizable that if an object is rocked two meters from the cot and it then stops, the child still tries to pull the cord. He even does the same thing in order to bring about the continuation of whistling, without seeing the adult who has produced it from behind a screen.

This primitive causality certainly verifies the fundamental idea of Maine de Biran, that initial causality is connected with action itself, but it verifies nothing else, for it is not at all the conscious realization of his self that leads the subject to discover causality, given that at this level there does not yet exist any differentiation between the self and the external world, and that the self will be constructed as a function of others only toward the first year and during the course of the following. It might be said that the consciousness of the self is unnecessary for the discovery of the causal relationship, but only for that of the voluntary effort, the resistances met and the centrifugal action

of one on the other. But let us first note that there is no awareness of a centrifugal stream of nervous impulses. Further, as far
as the voluntary effort and met resistances are concerned, nothing like it occurs. The child has grasped a cord and has observed
that this antecedent was followed by marvelous and unexpected
consequences and he has immediately begun again without
bothering about spatial and physical contacts (the case of the
object two meters away or of the whistling behind a screen). The
behavior of the child therefore conforms to the phenomenalism
of Hume, but only in the field of action itself, which verifies
Brunschvicg's observation that Hume and Maine de Biran refute each other. We will therefore speak of this first stage of
causality as magico-phenomenalist, phenomenalist because anything produces anything on the field of action, and magic because the action occurs independently of spatial and physical
contacts.

However, a concept is not understandable as a function of
its starting point alone, but only as a function of the whole of
its development, *i.e.* from the direction (or "intention"!) it
follows in its development. This consequence is striking: to the
extent that the child constructs the scheme of the permanent
object and organizes space as well as the temporal series according to a coherent system (the practical "group" of displacements), its causality becomes objectified and spatialized, that is
to say is extended to the relationships between the objects themselves and with a growing concern for contacts. In other words,
causality depends on a complete structuring of reality, due to
the development of intelligence, which on the whole verifies
the rationalist interpretation of causality in terms of inferential
construction, as against the phenomenalist one of Hume and
the intuition of an experienced passage between the cause and
effect of Maine de Biran.

However, this verification would be incomplete if there was
not a sequel. On the level of representative thought, from two
to eleven to twelve years, we observe, according to rule, a reconstruction of that which was acquired on the sensori-motor level,

then a much more extended progress. Broadly speaking we can say that on this new level causality begins as on the sensori-motor level, by a direct assimilation of reality to the schemes of action. But, on the other hand, it is then decentered from this initial egocentrism so that it becomes assimilation to operations. This is something different even though the operation derives from action, and it finally gives rise to the concept of causality based on rational deduction. It will suffice to give two examples of causality by assimilation to action. First, an example which recalls in striking fashion the magico-phenomenalist causality of the cord attached to the roof of the cot. Up to about six years, a large number of children seen by us believe that the moon follows them, walks, runs or retraces its steps just as the subject does, waits for him when he enters a house and even reappears after a block of houses, when he goes to find out whether it will be seen again at the next crossroad. Next, a child of five years observed daily who discovers that the air is "made by the hand," *i.e.* that which may be produced by the hand in waving a branch like a fan (whence the wind produced by the trees when swaying, the dust or waves when rising, the clouds which in moving produce the wind and are then pushed by it as in the ἀυτιηερίστασις of Aristotle). As an example of causality by assimilation to operations, let us simply point out that as soon as the additive operations (addition of number or the sum of classes) are constructed toward seven to eight years, the child who up to then did not believe in the conservation of sugar once dissolved in water ("the taste will go like a smell," etc.), comes to accept the conservation of its substance, then its weight and finally its volume (measured by the displacement of the water level) by assuming that the small particles, visible while dissolving, become smaller and smaller and invisible, but that their sum remaining constant equals the total substance of the original piece of sugar, then its weight and its volume. This is certainly atomism due to the "metaphysics of the dust" as Bachelard so nicely put it, but resulting from the start from an operational composition instead of attaining it after an initial qualitative phase.

The psychogenetic study of causality thus no more verifies the Biranian analysis of causality than the psychology of conduct verifies his interpretation of effort. The direct intuition of the self is not therefore a valid form of knowledge on which one can base an idealist metaphysics.

(D) The philosophical psychology of Maine de Biran is above all concerned to refute empiricism and it would easily have succeeded in this if it had not fallen into the opposite extreme of an intuitionism much too reflective to be suited to achieve its object. Bergson's psychology has, in a different way, tried to contradict and to go beyond the empiricist associationism then fashionable in laboratory psychology, and it succeeded all the more easily because at the moment that *Données immédiates de la conscience* appeared, the same anti-associationist tendencies, the same notion of the "stream of consciousness" and the same pragmatic emphasis on the whole action in opposition to the static associations, are found in W. James and already to some extent in his teacher Peirce, who converted him to pragmatism. Although interested in religious questions and finally taking up a pragmatist philosophy that has nothing metaphysical about it and has all the characteristics of a "wisdom" (naturally in the American style, but we can neither blame James for not having been born in India nor for not having taught at Königsberg in the eighteenth century), W. James was the epitome of the scientific psychologist who founded a laboratory without being an enthusiastic experimentalist (but this may have been due to his not finding collaborators or assistants suited to his fertile imagination), and yet he always wanted to submit himself completely to the facts of experience. I do not suggest that James directly influenced Bergson and I have not even tried to verify this, which in any case is unimportant, for it often happens that at a turning point in science two or more thinkers produce the same ideas independently of one another. I only assert that Bergson's anti-associationist ideas, his views on the temporal stream of consciousness and on the role of action cannot be attributed to his metaphysical intentions, since they are to be met from that time onward among writers wishing to revitalize scientific psychology. It is, on the contrary, with more specific ideas from the metaphysical point of view on the properties of the mind irreducible to those of the body that the Bergsonian theses begin to become questionable.

To return to the part played by action (see Chapter Three under C4), Bergson has admirably described the way in which perception divides up reality according to a rough outline of possible or projected actions, and which intelligence uses to extend action. But what is curious and in quite close parallelism with American pragmatism, is that he has looked at action from the point of view of its results and successes without referring to its preliminary and in some sort epistemological conditions, so that he has not even stressed the coordination of actions nor seen that this coordination involved a logic preparatory to that of the operations themselves, which are actions internalized and become reversible. He has certainly seen and brilliantly described the role of "anticipatory schemes" that direct the solution of a problem. This is probably a contribution that can with justice be placed to the credit of introspection, in a thinker moreover who had reflected much on the conditions of scientific invention. But he has not derived from it a general theory of schemes of action, which might have led him to stress the aspect of coordination and not only that of anticipation and of success. It is therefore not without such limiting reasons that he has arrived at the view according to which knowledge of life ought to turn away from action instead of making use of its epistemological presuppositions.

Let us now come to the metaphysical ideas of Bergsonian psychology, *i.e.* to the "innermost self" based on the analysis of the two memories, and the way in which it makes use of the body without it being located in the latter. This general conception starts, as one knows, from the analysis of the two memories: habit-memory and image-memory. Such a distinction is well-founded, in the sense that it could already be based on precise facts and has not been invalidated, since provided, as Janet has noted, that we only see in it a difference of level.[10] But each of the two terms thus distinguished calls for comments that considerably reduce the scope of the interpretations Bergson wished to derive from them.

Habit-memory, from the first, is not restricted to the sole function of repetition but also exhibits the fundamental one of "recognition." If Bergson had had a general theory of schemes of action, he would have seen that every scheme of assimilation that allows an action to be transposed in partially similar and partially novel situations in relation to the initial action, is at the same time the origin of repetition, of recognition, and of generalization. It follows that Bergson's two memories correspond to the two terms of the classic distinction between recognition memory, which is very primitive and occurs even among the lower invertebrates, and recollection of memory, of a very much higher level and which, in man, only appears with language, the mental image, etc., and in a general fashion with the semiotic (or symbolic) function.

As for recollection memory, or image-memory, Bergson accepts here one of two possible theses, without even mentioning or discussing the other. Let A be an event, then forgotten or about which the subject no longer thinks, but which at a later date is recalled under a form A′ once or several times. Two problems then arise: Is the memory-image A′ a faithful representation of A, and above all what has happened in the interval? Either A′, as soon as it is formed after the completion of A, has been stored as such in the subject's "unconscious," or A′ has vanished in the interval but has been reconstructed at the time of recall by means of a set of inferences reminiscent of the historian's reconstruction. Bergson and Freud adopt the first hypothesis, Janet adopts the second, making recollection memory one kind of "conduct" like any other "that of the narrative,"

[10] And consequently we need to take into account all the intermediaries between these levels. In work in progress on memory with B. Inhelder, we distinguish nine different types intermediate between habit-memory and the memory-image.

which consists in reconstructing and ordering the narrated events.

The second thesis has a greater probability of being true. What certainly remains in the "unconscious," or more precisely in the nonreflective behavior of the subject, is the totality of his schemes of action that aid the reconstruction. Let us ask someone who does not follow a regular routine if he had his breakfast before putting on his tie or afterward; he will be unable to answer, since it is unlikely that either one or the other of these two minor events have left images of the form A', and that these images, even if recorded in the "unconscious," are not themselves serially related in time. It is the reconstruction that introduces this seriation and often with great difficulty: for example, if one is asked to state whether one had had a second child before or after the coming of Fascism in Italy, before or after having written such a work, etc. If the same person is asked whether he has breakfasted before or after awakening he will reply straightaway, but by inference starting from schemes of action.

In support of the second thesis we particularly need to refer to the distorting character of some childhood memories. My earliest memory goes back to the time when I was still being pushed by a nurse in a pram; which would be a very exceptional memory if it were authentic. A man had tried to kidnap me but the nurse bravely defended me, being severely scratched as a result, and the man ran away when a policeman came up. This memory remains very vivid: I see again the whole scene, which took place at the roundabout of the Champs-Élysées. I still see the spectators who gathered and the arrival of the policeman with his short cape, which the police then wore, etc. When I was fifteen, the former nurse wrote to my parents saying that as she had been recently converted she wanted to confess her past faults. She had made up the story of the child who was nearly kidnapped, the scratches were faked, etc., and she returned the watch that had been given to her as a reward by my parents. This childhood memory is therefore one reconstructed visually (and this point is important), but starting from a story heard no doubt between five and ten years. If the memory were "true" in the sense of conforming to the events, it would nonetheless be reconstructed.

The part played by reconstruction and inference seems therefore to be very great in recollection memory, even if some memories are conserved. This fact alone somewhat undermines the thesis of a mind whose proper existence, considered as distinct from the body, would be connected with the complete conservation of the whole of its past history. It is true that one can conceive a third thesis according to which it would conserve more memories than those of which recall is possible. The latter then consists in a reconstruction, at least partial, of the inferential type, the two aspects of conservation and reconstruction remain thus in part independent. But even admitting this compromise, there is no proof that the forgotten memories are when stored purely mental and independent of the brain, as Bergson thinks. Recent experiments of W. Penfield have shown that if the temporal lobes of the brain are electrically stimulated, the subject can be made to relive with extraordinary vividness past scenes and at their natural rate, as in the case of a musical theme performed by orchestra and singer. In some of these relived experiences, the onlooker is himself the actor as in a dream, in others the states are still vivid but recalled as past, and finally in others there is no longer *aesthesia* but a situation comparable to that of the ordinary mental image.

One has some difficulty, moreover, in grasping the psychological meaning of the "innermost self" of Bergson, who, turning away from action and social life, would only find himself again in states close to dreams. It is difficult to see how these states could be distinguished from incoherent and schizoid ones.

But the main difficulty of the idealist psychology at which Bergson has ended, lacking a logic of action, is, being given the failure of the theory of a pure memory independent of the body, its negation of the principle of psycho-physiological parallelism. Consciousness is certainly not an epiphenomenon, since it consists in a system of meanings interconnected together by implicatory relationships, which excludes any reduction of consciousness to physical causality. Equally—but this is an entirely different question—mental life constantly influences the organism, as is proved by what in some quarters is called psychosomatic and in others cortico-visceral medicine, but it concerns the whole of mental life including the brain, and this does not at all prove that consciousness as such acts on matter: for matter comprises mass, force, forms of energy, extension, etc. In order for consciousness to act causally it would also need to possess these properties, which would give it a material form and make it lose its distinctive qualities. If we were therefore able to show in some definite instance the action of "mental energy," as Bergson puts it, on a region of matter, we would be led to distinguish immediately, within this energy, its causal aspect as, for example, that force overcomes a resistance, and its conscious aspect qua meanings, of such a kind that the problem would arise once again of the parallelism between the two aspects, the first being physical and the second conscious.

(E) The problem of mind and body plays an important part in an entirely different sense in the philosophical psychology of Merleau-Ponty because, restricted to the analysis of consciousness (including therein that latent consciousness which is the unconscious), but interested in the question of the body as represented by consciousness and in that of behavior as "embodied subjectivity," it finds itself constantly at grips with the central difficulty of phenomenology. This difficulty consists in having to explain everything by starting from an absolute beginning within consciousness, when all consciousness has a history which connects it with the schematism of action and by that to the organism.

Where Sartre sees only antithesis and magic, Merleau–Ponty, much superior by his permanent concern to reconcile ontology and epistemology, is constantly seeking for the originary experience which will provide this synthesis. But as there is certainly no such originary experience, and as Merleau-Ponty, distrusting all deduction, is no system builder, the whole of his psychology ends in stressing the "ambiguities" of consciousness up to its movement of "transcendence," which transforms a factual situation into an existence possessing meaning.

As Husserl's phenomenology claims to be an analysis not of "facts" but of "forms" of consciousness attaining objects, the latter remaining inseparable from the very act of consciousness, which gives them a "meaning" or connects them "intentionally," there are two possible ways of arriving at such an analysis, in some respects close to that of Kantianism, but with the added merit of remaining on the field of phenomena and of recognizing that the relations between subject and object were indissociable. These are the diachronic approach, *i.e.* historical and genetic, connecting these "forms," "intentions," or "meanings" to the schemes of action, which does not at all abolish "acts of consciousness" but leads us to give up subjectivity as the sole field of analysis; and the synchronic or static approach, which limits itself solely to subjectivity in order to find within it the originary experiences that would antedate the beginnings of knowledge. Husserl has chosen this second method, and it has finally led him to the hypothesis of a lived world or *Lebenswelt*, prior to all reflection and matrix of all knowledge. But as knowledge and its "forms" are not contained in advance in this originary experience, which only provides its starting point, and a series of other forms, intentions, and meanings are continuously elaborated, one can ask whether this is a real starting point, and whether it is not because the method used restricts one to the sphere of subjectivity that one is forced to postulate such an absolute beginning.

Merleau-Ponty's approach is similar, but it is much more paradoxical as he does not construct an epistemology or a general ontology like Husserl, but tries to reconstruct a psychology in which the historical or genetic dimensions and the connections with the body or behavior, as well as with the social world, are much more suggestive. As a consequence subjectivity, on which this more restricted but more concrete structure is based, is burdened with enormous tasks. Husserl's ablest commentator, E. Fink, has shrewdly noted that the central problem of the master is not that of Kant: "How is knowledge possible?" but a much vaster problem: How is the world possible, including therein knowledge? As long as it concerns the whole world this is acceptable, but as soon as it is a question of the human body and society, *i.e.* of behavior taken as a whole of which consciousness seems to be only an aspect, it appears futile to attempt to find within the primitive experience of the latter that which will explain all the rest.

Confining himself at first to knowledge, Merleau-Ponty holds that "the whole universe of science is constructed on the lived world," [11] therefore on this originary experience prior to all reflection and given in perception, while saying at the same time that science has not the same significance as this lived immediacy since it forms "a determination or an explanation" of it. There is therefore a construction proceeding from the lived to the reflective and it is then necessary to ask why should not the "lived" be itself "constructed" instead of being originary.

More precisely, two serious questions immediately arise. Firstly, is the "lived" the same for all subjects? If this is not the case, how can we derive from an individual subjectivity data enabling us to say something valid about the intentions or meanings giving rise to the epistemological subjectivity? If, on the contrary, this is the case, or if there are at least some elements common to the originary experiences of all subjects (and one asks for proof, but without seeing from where it could come except from the subjectivity itself), the second problem is to understand how this common structure originates. The Kantian *a priori* proceeds from a universal necessity, but such experience has neither an *a priori* nor necessary character, since it is given before all reflection and is to be found only on the phenomenal level. To say that we discover it there is no answer for someone who wishes to combat empiricism. We have then to extend our inquiry to the child and the animal, but what would then be-

[11] *Phénoménologie de la perception*, p. 11 (1945 edition).

come of the common elements and how can we extend our inquiry without referring to onto- or phylo-genetic mechanisms?

There is not the least proof that the lived world constitutes an originary experience, and the first question to ask regarding its position in the very logic of the doctrine is how this experience is possible; *i.e.* what are the preliminary conditions enabling it to give "meanings" (to objects, acts, etc.)? To bring in consciousness is not sufficient, for consciousness cannot be compared to a searchlight that reveals a world of readymade meanings or intentions already directed to objects. The characteristic feature of a meaning is to be relative to other meanings, *i.e.* to involve a *minimum* of system or organization. How does this system arise? From a series of acts that are neither discontinuous nor uncoordinated, without which there would be neither system nor meanings. To speak of intuition is understandable (but as such unacceptable) if it is a question of attaining in an immediate fashion nontemporal "essences," but we are within the lived, *i.e.* within the global relationship of the subject to perceived objects and the meanings are not therefore all given, otherwise the whole of knowledge would be performed in this original contact. For meaning to occur a series of acts is thus necessary, which are neither fortuitous nor completely deducible from each other from the start: in other words, if lived experience has a "meaning" it therefore has a history. The problem may be summed up as follows: at a time t, does the subject's lived experience depend only on this history to the extent in which this subject is conscious of his earlier development, at times $t - n$ or, on the contrary, is consciousness influenced by his history independently of the consciousness of this history? In other words, does consciousness contain within itself its own history or is it history (independently of the consciousness that depends on it) which contains consciousness? I believe that even if we agree with the phenomenologist that the whole of the subject's past history has always been conscious (which I would, of course, not admit), it will be difficult to maintain that the subject's consciousness at a time *t* is only influenced by his history if he knows it.

In a lecture at the *Rencontres internationales* of Geneva in 1951, Merleau-Ponty has accepted much of Freudianism while greatly reducing and rightly so the barrier between the conscious and unconscious. If one recognizes the importance of a genetic development in the case of affectivity, there is no reason for not doing the same for thought, and I readily go along with Merleau-Ponty when he argues, believing to contradict me, that the thought of the child subsists under that of the adult, provided one admits that there has been a transformation and construction from the first to the second.

As soon as one accepts the fact that consciousness has a history and the existence of historical influences of which one is not completely conscious, the problem of lived experience prior to all reflection arises in completely different terms. What is of importance in it is no longer its content, which can vary from individual to individual, but its general capacity to form intentions and give meanings which therefore presupposes an organization since the latter are relative to each other. This organization must not be taken as *a priori*, which would bring us back to Kant. It is important only to note that by connecting together meanings (and they are necessarily connected) diachronically and moreover synchronically, the subject is necessarily involved in assimilations and differentiations. He thus constructs a schematism, as dynamic and bound up with its content as one would wish for, but a schematism nonetheless, and which occurs from perception onward: for the *Gestalten* are schemes and are not discontinuously re-created at the time of each situation or object analogous to the preceding ones. And it occurs from action onward: for the repetition of an action in similar circumstances is not a matter of an associative mechanism, but of meanings due to schemes of assimilation which ensure this generalization.

We are, therefore, whether we like it or not, faced with the central question of the relations between consciousness and behavior. Merleau-Ponty refers to the latter as "embodied subjec-

M

tivity" because it is imbued with intention and meaning. But the same problem is found again: Is consciousness influenced by the history of this behavior only to the extent in which it actually includes this history in a total apperception? If the answer is affirmative, it effectively directs the whole of actual behavior; if negative, it only partially directs it and remains partially subordinated to a schematism in which the action of which the lived experience, despite its apparent immediacy, only forms a more or less adequate conscious realization. Merleau-Ponty, moreover, recognizes that "one does not act with the mind alone" and with K. Goldstein stresses the unity of the organism in its physiological and mental functions. But if this is true, it implies both that consciousness is not everything, and that for the concept of consciousness considered as a primary fact, it is necessary to substitute the dynamism of "conscious realizations" in which we perceive at first the intentions and results of acts before being able to grasp their complete mechanism, that is to say the schematism arising from the linking of earlier acts. As soon as we place ourselves at the point of view of functional totalities, and as soon as we reintroduce the historical dimension from which they are inseparable, we no longer have the right to speak of the originary experiences of lived consciousness. For they are neither primitive, since they have a past, nor completely adequate as conscious realizations, since they fail to take account of an important part of the underlying schematism that makes them possible.

Similar remarks apply to the question of "intersubjectivity." Merleau-Ponty fully recognizes, with Husserl, that subjectivity is intersubjective, and he also rightly stresses the very process by which intersubjectivity occurs as one of dialectical development. But he only knows intersubjectivity as reflected in each subjectivity. The same problem only then arises here as in connection with consciousness and its history, since the process by which intersubjectivity occurs is one of historical development: Is the subject only influenced by the totality of social interactions to the extent in which he is conscious of them, or do these interactions in their diachronic and even synchronic functioning go beyond consciousness? And if they do, as is evident, how can we from this point of view still believe that lived experience can be originary?

But if the search for originary experiences forms one of the two fundamental aspects of the thought of Merleau-Ponty, and if it can only lead to an *impasse* as soon as the historical or dialectical dimension is restored, the other aspect is, on the contrary, the analysis of the process of "transcendence" by which consciousness constructs new meanings and proceeds from the "intentionality of the act" (or thetic) to "operative intentionality," which will finally lead to intellectual consciousness in creating existences by ascribing meaning to what are only factual situations. Let us frst note that Merleau-Ponty has certainly felt the latent contradiction between these two positions, for if there is a dialectical process generating new meanings, how are we to conceive the initial "thetic intentions" without ascribing to them the prior "operative intentions"? This is certainly what he comes to assume near the end of the *Phénoménologie de la perception,* in glimpsing the existence of an "art hidden in the depths of the human soul and which, like all art, is only known through its results." In less well-chosen words, this is exactly what we call the schematism of action, of which so-called immediate conscious experience only knows the resultants! But this latent contradiction between the willingness to consider lived experience as originary and the capacity then given to it of indefinitely transcending itself has a more serious consequence than the incompletion of a system. It leads to this result, which, it must be acknowledged, Merleau-Ponty has brought out into the light of day instead of trying to hide it, that in not trying to get outside subjectivity and in considering the "historical situation," the body and behavior, merely in the perspective of this subjectivity, one only discovers "ambiguities." Where the anti-intellectualism of Sartre sees "magic" everywhere, that of Merleau-Ponty discovers ambiguities, which is already much more rational. But we still have to see whether this "ambiguity" belongs to the system or to reality.

Of course it belongs to both, *i.e.* to the way in which the system has divided up reality so as to retain only subjectivity, and Merleau-Ponty's description of the latter is at once very profound in that in fact subjectivity is ambiguous, and very biased because it is incomplete, it being given that subjectivity is not everything. "Philosophical" psychology constantly criticizes scientific psychology for not ending in an "anthropology" able to express the whole of man, and I have in particular been constantly criticized for being an intellectualist because I am only interested in cognitive functions. In the perspective of such discussions, let us recognize that the result of this work, alas incomplete, is all the same saddening, from which there only emerges in the state in which it has been left a picture of man as an ambiguous consciousness. No, the distinctive feature of man is not that of being a subjectivity: it is constantly to accomplish a task, a *praxis* as Marxism puts it, or "works" as I. Meyerson said, and to do it consciously but above all effectively because consciously tending toward a result. To accomplish a task is to start from data as objective as possible in order to end at results as objective as possible, and if objectivity is only an ideal or a limit, it is all the same one of the fundamental dimensions of human "intentionality." To tell us that "I am here and now" is "ambiguous" because I am already elsewhere is a philosophical joke, for it is not at all ambiguous as soon as I know where I want to go. It matters little that from the point of view of subjectivity all "intention," all "existence," etc., is ambiguous. They are only ambiguous if one regards them as such by dividing them up artificially, but they cease to be so if they are connected to the general coordination of actions, origin of rational activity, and of the objective result aimed at, which is to modify external reality in turning away from the "self," which is the only specific object of study for philosophical psychology.

(F) Let us then conclude. We have compared four important "philosophical psychologies." We have seen the failure of

Maine de Biran's analysis of effort and of causality because he centered them on the "self." We have seen how Bergson has neglected action, the cognitive importance of which he had, however, stressed in order to look for the "innermost self" in the irrational setting of the dream. We have seen Sartre project his self into consciousness in general in order to discover there that its "causality" is magic, and we see Merleau-Ponty end by concluding that subjectivity is basically ambiguous. This is, then, what is given to us as knowledge of Man and which is opposed to the psychology of conduct, because the latter is intellectualist and only "scientific."

The reasons for such a failure are very plain and we have already noted them. One can be interested in subjectivity and introspection as much as one pleases; this is not the distinctive mark of philosophical psychology, since the experimental psychologists can be concerned just as much with them according to the problems they study. For example, P. Fraisse in order to study temporal conduct needs introspective data, among others, and because he has described the methods and praised the progress of scientific psychology in our *Traité de psychologie expérimentale* this does not mean that he ignores such facts. Only when the psychologist uses them he tries to arrive at an "objective" interpretation, if we may put it thus, for despite unconsciously or consciously entertained misunderstandings, "objective" does not always mean "he who neglects the subject" but always "he who tries to avoid the illusions of his self" in studying methodically the reactions of others. On the other hand, the striking character of philosophical introspection is that it relies simply on its own honesty and virtuosity of analysis as guarantees of truth, as if sincerity and ability enabled one to avoid systematic errors. The result is that, like all general metaphysical systems, philosophical "psychologies" are above all the reflection of a personality. In adopting as an exclusive method not only introspection, which by itself is deceptive if unrelated to conduct, but introspection centered exclusively on one's "self," however inspired it may be, they cannot dissociate the general philosophy of the part of the self that observes and the data inherent in the other part of the self, which is only supposed to be observed when one dictates to it in varying degrees the answers to be given.

The seriousness of this misunderstanding not only depends on the question of method, which is already very serious; it depends just as much on the fact that we do not perceive its nature and that we make what is only a question of method a dispute about theories. There is absolutely nothing in the hypotheses of the philosophical psychologies we have discussed that is in itself a priori contrary to a scientific position, because a science is only valid if it is open. T. Flournoy, a good psychologist who had already described the unconscious in quasi-Freudian terms at the beginning of 1900 (before the Traumdeutung) based his research on two principles: (1) everything is possible ("there are more things in heaven and earth than in all our philosophy"); but (2) the weight of evidence ought to be proportional to the strangeness of the facts (and I would add myself: to the more or less personal character of their initial observation). That the self be a force in the sense of Maine de Biran. Why not? That there exist originary live experiences from which knowledge derives, or privileged "intuitions," that psychological "causality" is irrational, etc. Everything is possible, and this is not the question here. But when under the pretext of reacting against positivism, objectivism, etc., personal philosophical theses are put forward as being the true psychology, this is to scorn the rules of the game and to confuse the study of subjectivity in general with the championing of personal subjectivity.

Philosophers and
Problems of Fact

Chapter Five

THIS FINAL CHAPTER adds nothing to the discussion of principles
in Chapters Two to Four, but it seems to me to be useful by
way of supporting evidence, although it only deals with examples
selected somewhat at random. The problem is the following.
The three main fields that deal with the problems of knowledge
are those of norms, facts, and intuition. It is perfectly natural
for philosophers to deal with the question of norms, for if we try
to deal with problems of principles and foundations, we are
forced to discuss norms. Logic is the science of formal truth, and
a logical demonstration must be accepted. But these formal
norms need to be coordinated with the totality of problems, and
it is therefore natural that reflection should be concerned with
these questions of coordination. Intuition, on the other hand, is,
for those believing in it, a direct grasping of the object and gives
us truth, *i.e.* it is both normative and ontological or factual. The
ideal of a mode of knowledge peculiar to philosophy therefore
always involves an appeal to intuition, and hence it is once again
normal that philosophy concerns itself with intuitive knowledge.
There remains, on the contrary, problems of fact, and in this
respect two positions are possible.

The first is that of intuitionist philosophies like phenomenology, which does not claim to deal with facts, which are the
concern of science, but only with "forms," which these facts
presuppose, therefore with intentions and meanings, etc., or, in
short, with essences. From such a point of view conflict is inevitable with any form of knowledge having a scientific char-

acter. For psychology an intention and a meaning are still facts, and the "reduction" proceeding from the spatio-temporal to extratemporal concepts is still a fact—a fact being by definition that which is studied when we decenter our inquiries in relation to the self. It is pointless to return to this problem discussed in Chapter Three.

On the other hand, contemporary philosophers who use reflective or dialectical methods, without restricting themselves to the conceptual apparatus of phenomenological ontology, constantly refer to questions of fact, since they are interested in reality as a whole and not only in formal logic. So also do the phenomenologists, if only to distinguish facts and essences. We have seen (Chapter Four under B) how Sartre, for example, regarded facts as a collection of accidents. We then need to examine how philosophers deal with questions of fact, especially as the whole of their training only enables them to deal with their problems in a purely reflective manner, while a fact presupposes at the least a process of verification, and this can only be carried out if one has some definite method.

To my knowledge only one contemporary philosopher has dealt with this problem of method, apart, of course, from the philosophers of science, who have studied the nature of facts in experimental science: for example, the admirable analysis of G. Bachelard in La connaissance approchée. But this is another question; what we ask here is, what do philosophers do when in their studies and independently of all theories of experience or of experimental method they have to refer to facts. The only philosophy that seems to have taken this problem seriously is the "idonéisme" of F. Gonseth, a philosopher of science, it is true, but one who is not afraid of discussing general questions as, on occasion, that of freedom. Among the principles introduced by Gonseth at the beginning of his philosophy, like that of openness, is one of which little note has been taken, because in its context it appears to be self-evident. It is that of "technicality," according to which all knowledge is relative to the use of a particular technique that alone guarantees it, for example, axiomatic formalization in the case of deductive knowledge, or the different types of methodical observation (with the use of statistical controls) or experimentation in the case of knowledge of facts. As the use of every technique requires some previous training, Gonseth concludes that the only valid facts that philosophers ought to refer to are those established by specialists, which seems self-evident.

But before seeing how little this is true for a large number of philosophers, let us first try to understand why it is so much more difficult to arrive at a valid fact than a correct deduction. Experimental physics began more than twenty centuries after mathematics and logic, and another two centuries has been needed before it has been realized that psychology presupposes experimentation. The reasons for this are of a twofold kind, subjective and objective. Objectively, a fact can only be arrived at by systematically isolating the factors involved, and it required the genius of a Galileo to study successfully simple motions when the movements of everyday observation, like the fall of a leaf, are often of an inextricable complexity. As against this, logico-mathematical deduction starts immediately from simple operations like class-inclusion, the starting point of the syllogistic, or the addition of integers. In the case of psychology the isolation of factors is still much more complex, since they are organically related together into wholes difficult to vary systematically. I will always remember the surprise and admiration I felt in listening to Einstein at Princeton, who liked to be told the facts of child psychology (particularly the nonconservations), when he invariably concluded: "How difficult it is! How much more difficult psychology is than physics!" But one needs to be Einstein in order to grasp so quickly a difficulty that few people understand, and unfortunately not always the psychologists themselves. . . .

Subjectively, the difficulty in studying facts as against everyday deductive inferences (I do not speak of deduction in pure mathematics or in mathematical physics) is because it is much more economical to reflect and to deduce than to experiment.

One of P. Janet's discoveries, when he tried to construct stages of mental development, basing it not on the child but on the hierarchy of functions in psychopathology (according to their complexity and expenditure of necessary energy), was to replace the reflective stage below that of the stage where the "sense of reality" makes systematic work and experimentation possible. He pointed out that the psychasthenics and the anxiety prone reflect easily and even too much, while their sense of reality is disturbed the power to reflect, which remains unaffected is hence increased. In the child the first concrete deductions begin toward seven-eight years, reflection in Janet's sense (with the possibility of reasoning about hypotheses and no longer only about objects) toward eleven to twelve years, and the first experimental forms of conduct with the systematic isolation of factors only toward fourteen to fifteen years. We know how they are then lost in most of the liberal professions, when they are not kept up at the university; and this because of the lack, at least in my country, of any education for a second degree in which the experimental approach is encouraged, which nevertheless occurs spontaneously in the child.[1]

Let us now return to philosophy, first noting that in many countries there is a marked increase in the number of philosophers as compared with earlier centuries when philosophy was not a profession but an exceptional achievement. It might be said that the same thing has happened with scientists. However, a mediocre scientist can still carry out useful work in a limited field, while an undistinguished philosopher is a little like an untalented artist or novelist. If then philosophy is concerned with reality as a whole, it is assumed to be possible to train specialists in this complete knowledge or search for the absolute, without their first having had some training in the field of partial or relative knowledge. It is true that they have acquired a sense

[1] See B. Inhelder and J. Piaget, *De la logique de l'enfant à la logique de l'adolescent*, Paris, Presses Universitaires de France, 1955. (English translation, *The Growth of Logical Thinking from Childhood to Adolescence*, Basic Books, 1958).

of history and a respect for texts, since the only specialization demanded of them is the history of philosophy, but as far as methods of knowledge are concerned, only reflection is used, which, moreover, corresponds to the deep-rooted tendencies of adolescence and the natural inclination of the human mind. Hence, when they have not the exceptional courage to specialize in the epistemology of a particular science and to advance knowledge of the latter, as has been the case with Cavailles, Lautmann, and Vuillemin in mathematics, G. and S. Bachelard in physics, Daudin and F. Meyer in biology, C. G. Granger in economics and social science, L. Goldmann in sociology, etc., the studies engaged in by philosophers are either historical, or reflective in the most general sense. In such a situation, the knowledge of facts is divorced from that which alone can give it the character of knowledge properly so called, that is to say, from an inquiry into its technicality. There is therefore a strong temptation, moreover, under an unconscious or implicit form, to assume that reflection on fact is, in this case, subsequent and not prior to the establishment of fact (since, in the event, the latter has already in general been established by others), that it is of a higher order than the latter and consequently can intervene actively in the interpretation of fact, rectifying and completing it where necessary.

We must not therefore be surprised to see philosophers at all levels, meddling in physics in order to challenge the theory of relativity, in biology to challenge evolution or to reinterpret it in their own manner in order to solve problems of finality and sometimes of structure, and above all intervening in psychology or sociology and in all the human sciences.

(A) In the field of physics the theory of relativity has stimulated in the highest degree the reflections of philosophers, but in two very different ways. The steadfast position of L. Brunschvicg, which is well known, is that the task of philosophy is not to concern itself with questions of fact, arising solely from technical and specialist disciplines, but to ask in the Kantian manner how this knowledge has become possible. His attitude toward relativity is therefore not to question it, but only one of epistemological reflection: whence his excellent account of the new mode of interaction between the measuring instrument and the measured which the relativistic coordination presupposes, or between the spatio-temporal container and the physical content, the former ceasing to be a dissociable framework so as to become an aspect of this content itself. It has been possible to be deceived here because of the endless ambiguity of the individual subject and the epistemological subject. A. Metz, overlooking that measuring operations involve the whole activity of the subject, in the second sense of the term, believed he had refuted this interpretation by noting that measurements are the concern of meter rods and clocks effectively modified by the fields in which they are placed, as if Brunschvicgian "idealism" maintained the opposite and reduced the subject to a set of "mental images" (these are Metz's words). Brunschvicg's intention is not at all to modify the relativistic data: but only to show how the interactions between the operational activity of the subject and experience, much more restricted than was assumed before Einstein, ought to lead to such a revival of epistemological inquiry.

But for other philosophers, on the contrary, the theory of relativity, in attacking the most general problem of whether time and space were absolute or not, has seemed to involve an immediate encroachment upon the very field of philosophy and consequently to authorize a discussion on this common ground and on equal terms, as if the physicist, in challenging the existence of an absolute up to then accepted as such, gave the philosopher *ipso facto* the right to intervene in the field of physics. On this point, the motives are not always the same, and it might be interesting to distinguish them. I have mentioned in Chapter One how my excellent teacher A. Reymond had formed the project of refuting Einsteinian theory. He had no imperialistic pretensions nor any philosophical arrogance, and he was the first to laugh at such formulae as "philosophy tells us that . . . ," imbued as he was by the idea that the different philosophical positions could never be reduced to each other. But he had his beliefs, and the fact that an absolute had tottered caused him a veritable moral anxiety of such a sort that without asking whether he was competent, which is secondary when there is a moral danger, he believed it his duty to defend a space and above all a time, which remained a little for him as for Newton a *sensorium Dei*. I imagine that in Maritain the conflict between relativity and Thomism is similarly motivated, but perhaps depends still more on a global opposition of these modes of thought. For Bergson, on the other hand, the situation is much more curious. Having opposed to psychological time relative to its own content and inseparable from it, a physical time conceived as spatialized and purely formal to a point where a general change of velocities would not at all alter it, Bergson was faced with the distressing situation of a new physics in which time was bound up with its content and its velocities, a time whose heterogeneous and real character recalls certain aspects of the Bergsonian duration! In place of renouncing his antithesis or modifying them, Bergson's reaction was—and this is of great interest for our purpose—to question the theory of relativity and to intervene on the basis of philosophical reflection alone in the technical discussion of the problem.

It would seem useless to labor Maritain's position (*Réflexions sur l'intelligence*, Paris, 1926, Chapters Five and Seven), since Thomism is a philosophy which in fact is always bound up with a religious faith, and that in such a case the "natural" powers attributed to reason and the "philosophy of nature" derivative from them are in reality prescribed in advance by a position taken up with respect to the supernatural. But as Aristotelianism is a philosophy of common sense, Maritain's trenchant and imperturbable dogmatism is of interest, since it expresses in the crudest form that which in fact corresponds to certain tendencies of every philosophy claiming to arrive at a form of knowledge independent of all science.

For Kantianism, which Maritain has seen expresses one of the fundamental aspects of modern science, *to know is to con-*

struct (p. 24). For realism, whose position he wishes to restore, to know "consists in being or becoming *the other insofar as it is the other*" (p. 53), therefore to identify oneself "immaterially" and "intentionally" with the object (cf. the *intentio* which, by the intermediary of Brentano, reappears in the Husserlian intuition). The power thus given to "natural" reason of placing itself directly in reality then leads one in all logic to give to common sense, guardian of this "reason," and consequently to the philosopher, who codifies and reflects the common reason he finds in himself and around him, the right and the duty of stating a certain number of general principles from which science itself would not be exempted, except to fall into sophism or into aberration. In a completely unambiguous table (p. 189) on "the division of the sciences," which we will discuss, Maritain divides them therefore into metaphysics ("Science of first principles speaking in absolute terms"), into mathematics (itself subject to mathematical philosophy or "Resolvent metaphysical science of the first principles of order" and quantity), and into physics, itself subject to the "Philosophy of nature." There is therefore a complete and continual subordination of science to metaphysics.

A first example clearly shows where this leads us: "It is thus . . . that the principle of inertia . . . arises from natural philosophy; and if the latter is forced to declare this principle unacceptable in the sense in which Descartes and Galileo understood it, it will be for positive science to revise the language in which it is expressed, and come to an agreement with philosophy" (p. 190, n.1). A second example of the "absurdity of philosophical thoughts carried along and expressed by the language" of science is that of the "event," which "occurred with Lobatchevsky, Riemann and metageometry" (p. 248). In other words, the philosopher is not satisfied, which would set a serious problem of legitimacy, to find a "basis" for science, leaving the scientist free to construct whatever structure he would wish on these preliminary foundations. The "philosophy of nature" as Maritain understands it, claims to enter immediately into every sort of technical discussion, and to correct the position of specialists on questions as vital for the future of science as the principle of inertia and the generalizations of geometry! It is small consolation for a psychologist, used to the intervention of some philosophers into his still insecure science, to find here a larger-than-life caricature of this imperialism, in the guise of a metaphysician who calmly attacks the basic principles of mechanics and general metric.

We can then guess what J. Maritain's reaction is to the theory of relativity. But it is not without interest, quite apart from the splendid presumptuousness of tone, for it amounts to a kind of nominalist Kantianism: the theory of relativity is scientifically acceptable as a "construction" of phenomena relative to the conventionally selected measurements, but behind these "appearances" described therefore in a valid fashion there remains the noumenon. The only slight difference from Kant is that here the noumenon can be grasped by "common sense," that is to say, speaking concretely, by caretakers and window-cleaners as well as the "philosophers of nature." This common sense therefore requires simultaneity at a distance and universal time, and it only remains to reinterpret Einstein's theories in order to make them compatible with this requirement of metaphysics and good sense combined.

The reconciliation is simple and consists in examining forthwith how the relativists have constructed their phenomena: it is "a physical measurement which a man would be able to make with his senses and his instruments under such or such conditions, moreover, as fanciful as one would wish, from the moment they are imaginable." "We have here," adds Maritain, "the fundamental principle, the philosophical rock, the holy of holies of the Einsteinian method" (p. 204). In other words, the theory of relativity is based on "nominal definitions" and has nothing to do with reality (p. 204): in defining simultaneity in an inadequate fashion (p. 208) it only attains an "apparent simultaneity" (p. 214), i.e. an "empirico-quantitative substitute. We are faced here with a breaking point between natural philosophy and physico-mathematical science. But no matter how this substitute be determined, as, for example, in Einstein's fashion, the essence of simultaneity itself still remains that which intelligence has conceived and defined" (p. 220). But physical measurement only proceeds by means of "accidental standards. What the thing measured is intrinsically and in its absolute dimensions (*sic*) cannot be determined by the Physicist" (p. 251). As for knowing what these "absolute dimensions" are, it is quite simply the "measured quantity with the standard belonging to nature—inaccessible to our Science"! (p. 251). Similarly, the relativistic invariants are looked for "on the wrong side of the common sense procedures," *i.e.* not from the side of "being" and "not within things," but "in the externality of quantitative relations which ought to remain the same from all possible points of view," etc. (p. 239).

The "absolute dimensions," the "standard of belonging to nature," the invariant looked for "within things," such are therefore the concepts of "natural philosophy" which Maritain opposes to those of Einstein. These gems of wisdom ought to be collected in a philosophical scrapbook for the use of future historians of thought. This does not prevent the metaphysician from concluding his chapter on Einstein's theories by seriously asserting: "Legitimate as scientific symbols . . . they are absurd when they are erected into philosophical expressions of reality. . . . In this case, they represent no more than a rather alarming symptom of the intellectual anarchism in which under the action of the disgraceful residues of Kantianism, and lacking a firm philosophical foundation modern science risks capsizing" (p. 259). It is worth giving these few quotations in order to show what becomes of the "legitimate symbols" of science in the light of the "philosophy of nature": a consistent language no longer expresses anything at all.

(B) Bergson's small book *Durée et simultaneité* (1922) is, of course, of a much higher standard, as far as the thought and language used. But it is surprising to note that underlying Bergson's tactfulness of expression, and once admitting the metaphysical differences between Bergsonism and Thomism, the arguments appealed to do not differ fundamentally.[2] Bergson did not see in the theory of relativity a nominalist Kantianism, "but we believe that it would be necessary to give this physics an idealistic interpretation, if we wished to make it into a philosophy" (p. 110, n.1). He does not say that the times relative to different observers are simple "appearances," but he speaks of times "attributed," or again "fictitious, imagined, computed," etc., in opposition to the only real time, which is that of the observer "living and conscious." "If . . . we accept Einstein's hypothesis the multiple times will subsist, but only one alone will ever be the real . . . : the others will be mathematical fictions" (p. 34). The only real time remains therefore lived time.

However, Bergson cannot fail to admit that this lived time depends partly on the environment, and this fact ought therefore to make him accept relative times and to see in them even a sort of extension of the Bergsonian duration (but this might have been at the price of sacrificing one of his fundamental antitheses): "Thus our duration and a certain experienced, lived participation of our material environment in this internal duration are facts of experience. . . . There is no rigorous proof that we will find the same durations when we change our environment: different durations, that is to say with different rhythms, would be able to co-exist. We have formerly made an hypothesis of this kind concerning living species" (p. 57). This passage then shows that we do not exaggerate when we speak of possible connections between Bergsonism and relativity. But Bergson refuses to extend them because "the nature of this participation is unknown: it might depend on a property which external things have, *without enduring themselves* [our italics] of manifesting themselves in our duration insofar as they act upon us . . . , etc." (p. 57). In other words, if the lived durations are relative to their content, physical time remains universal and empty and the relative times of Einstein simply occur there as

[2] I am not writing history here: Bergson's work is four years earlier than that of Maritain.

fictions originating from the fact that different possible observers for one and the same given time are imagined by a single real observer: "Reflection strengthens our conviction and even ends by making it unshakable, because it reveals to us in the Time of restricted Relativity—only one among them excepted —times without duration, in which events would not succeed each other, nor things subsist, nor beings age" (pp. 240–41).

This "unshakable conviction" due solely to philosophical "reflection" has, however, ended by Bergson giving way, since the last edition of the *Oeuvres complètes* of the Master produced according to his instructions, contains neither *Durée et simultaneité* nor any mention of this work. But this was not without difficulty. A. Metz published several articles in order to show Bergson's errors, but the latter replied coldly: ". . . he did not even suspect the difficulty. The meaning of my reflections including that of my book has completely escaped him. I cannot do anything about it." J. Becquerel wrote and went to see him, but in vain. Einstein in congratulating A. Metz on his book wrote (with permission to reproduce): "It is regrettable that Bergson so seriously deceives himself and his error is of a purely physical order, independent of all dispute between philosophical schools." E. Le Roy, the ablest disciple of Bergson, said in his turn in 1937: "As conceived from Bergson's point of view, a reference system has this strange character, nothing can be referred to it physically."

Bergson's encounter with relativity theory is highly instructive as far as the fate reserved for the interventions of philosophers in problems of facts are concerned, when they assume they have the right to discuss questions of the interpretation of experimental data and of computation. Bergson certainly tells us in his preface that he is not concerned with the "physical" aspect of the problem and that the "confusion" (p. vi) discovered by him only concerns the theory of relativity if one "makes it into a philosophy" (p. vii). But in a language more refined than that of Maritain, this once again comes to asserting that science does not attain reality, and that in order to achieve this it is necessary to remember that "science and philosophy are different disciplines, but made in order to complete themselves" (p. v), as if philosophy provided "knowledge" which imposed "the duty of bringing about a confrontation" (p. v). Without entering into this last discussion in its general form A. Metz, in a recent article (*Sciences*, 1964, no. 33, Hermann), limits himself to soberly stating: "Bergson's attitude of instructing the relativists as to what is (according to him) the theory of relativity may appear surprising. It occurs throughout the book. . . . The whole book is . . . full of statements as to 'the essence of the theory of relativity' and of that which one ought to do and say 'if one puts oneself at the point of view of relativity.' " Before Bergson finally listened to the voice of reason Einstein had to show in what he was "so badly mistaken." Now, Bergson's error raises precisely the problem with which the whole of our book is concerned, *i.e.* of the legitimacy of a "philosophical knowledge" distinct from scientific knowledge and able to correct it in factual detail. In connection with Langevin's space-capsule, Bergson has said, and it is here that he is mistaken: "We can only express ourselves mathematically on the hypothesis of a privileged system, even when we have begun by asserting reciprocity; and the physicist feeling no longer indebted to the hypothesis of reciprocity once he has paid lip service to it in arbitrarily selecting his reference system, leaves it to the philosopher and expresses himself henceforth in the language of the privileged system. Having faith in this physics Paul will enter the space-capsule. *En route* he will see that philosophy is right" (pp. 108–09). We have just seen how.

(C) If contemporary physics can still give rise to philosophical speculation despite its precise character and high degree of technicality, it goes without saying that in biology the situation appears to a large number of thinkers to call for a collaboration between scientific inquiry and metaphysics. The reasons for this are of two kinds.

The first is that biology has not yet solved its main problems.

Neither the mechanism of evolution nor the general structure of the organism is yet known, and without a mastery of these two perspectives, diachronic and synchronic, biology is at a stage comparable to that of physics before Newton, but with much more partial knowledge. It is therefore natural that philosophical speculation tries to fill the gap still left open by this present lack of possible syntheses. As this state of affairs is particularly favorable to such speculations, one cannot but believe it to be permanent because it is a feature of life. One therefore needs to have an uncommon philosophical courage to consider in connection with biology, not merely meta-biological solutions, but as F. Meyer has done, among others, in his *Problématique de l'évolution*, specifically epistemological analyses. In these analyses he has tried to distinguish levels of phenomena or levels of problems, in the hope of helping scientific inquiry itself and not its speculative substitutes.

The second reason is a more serious one and most instructive as far as the consequences of the contemporary organization of university studies are concerned. A biologist, in addition to his special branches of study, has studied chemistry, physics, and a little mathematics, particularly statistics, but he knows nothing about experimental psychology, linguistics, economics, etc., *i.e.* those sciences concerned with phenomena arising from living activities, which could suggest to him all kinds of models concerning processes raising problems of finality. With some exceptions, he is therefore unacquainted with information theory, decision theory (or game theory), and the details of cybernetic applications to questions of learning or intellectual adaptation. Consequently, he has thought little about the problem of structures as one meets them in general algebra, and in all that important region which today relates these questions of structure to those of probability. Leaving the field of his professional training, he has most chance of becoming acquainted with philosophy under its ordinary and general forms. When faced with the actual lacunae of his science as regards the basic problems of life, he either adopts an attitude which he calls mechanistic, and which in the final analysis attributes everything to chance, or a diametrically opposed attitude of favoring every general speculative interpretation, with which he has had practically no acquaintance in his actual studies, but which he finds intellectually satisfying enabling him to criticize the inadequacies of explanations in terms of chance. It is often a question of two successive periods in the same scientific career. I have, for example, followed with intense interest the evolution of the ideas of an eminent geneticist and specialist in the field of regeneration, E. Guyénet, as our continued acquaintance in the same Faculty enabled me to question him often. During the first period, Guyénet was only interested in the ideas of chance and selection in the Neo-Darwinian manner. I objected that all psychological explanation would thus become impossible, and that if his own brain was the product of successive random events with subsequent approximate selections all theory becomes singularly tenuous. He invariably replied that giving up chance would mean introducing finalism, which he personally had decided "to oppose," that psychology is of no interest to the biologist, since it is "philosophy," and that such a point of view introduces finalism. From this all-or-none position Guyénet has then reaped the consequences the day when he ceased to believe in the explanatory value of chance. Having become a finalist and a quasi-vitalist, he no better understood why I did not follow him, as if there existed nothing between a so-called mechanism reducing itself to a random selection and the Aristotelian philosophy of finality. However, in this same Faculty the physicist C. E. Guye developed the most profound ideas on the frontiers of physics and biology, showing that if classical physical chemistry is unable to integrate vital phenomena, this integration seems nearer with the changes occurring in microphysics and will enrich the latter with new dimensions instead of impoverishing the complexity of the organism. C. E. Guye even generalized this nonreduction interpretation, but by reciprocal assimilation, foreseeing a more "general" [3] physico-chemistry which will integrate cerebral activities.

The present instability of biological positions, which as far as the important problems are concerned, oscillate between inadequate explanatory schemes and facile speculation, encourages the claims of a parascientific psychology ever willing to complete the lacunae of science. Where, we may ask, will such enterprises lead? We merely give two examples. The first is not a new one, but it is of interest, since R. Dalbiez, the philosopher who puts forward these theses, asked several distinguished biologists to discuss the facts, leaving the general conclusions for himself. He considers that "there are at the present time few tasks more pressing that the reconstitution of a philosophy of nature." [4] He wanted this philosophy to be the product of a collaboration between philosophers and scientists. It is therefore interesting to see what this collaboration has produced.

The book *Le transformisme*, which attempts to answer this question, begins with an essay by E. Gagnebin showing the reasons given by paleontology for believing in evolution without as such arriving at the causes of the latter. As against this, L. Vialleton states his well-known reservation on evolutionism, by suggesting a return to Cuvier. W. R. Thomson shows the difficulty of explaining the parasitic forms by the disuse of organs, and stresses the existence of useful variations while carefully specifying the limits of finalistic interpretations in which he believed, but on the condition of not making them account for the detail. L. Cuénot finally refutes every hypothesis of a transmission of acquired characteristics, without as yet maintaining this "modified finalism, restricted or intermittent, expressing itself by the perfectible invention," which he later [5]

[3] Guye believed that in physics it is the complex and not the simple which enables us to make true generalizations, for example, electro-magnetism as against classical mechanics.

[4] *Le transformisme* by L. Cuénot, R. Dalbiez, E. Gagnebin, W. R. Thomson and L. Vialleton, Vrin, 1927, p. 218.

[5] L. Cuénot, *Invention et finalité en biologie*, Flammarion, 1941, p. 246.

opposed to explanations by chance alone. In short, the four contributions brought together by Dalbiez are models of prudence, expressing objectively enough the difficulty of the problems.

We then get the philosopher's conclusion. Science, he concedes, has for its object "the external world, while reserving for philosophy this final explanation of matter and life" (p. 202). But Dalbiez, while offering this "final" explanation, discusses no less energetically actual facts, which he therefore in no way considers as "reserved" by reciprocity for science. He accepts transformism, but notes the absence of any distinction between "types" and their variations, the former "never being considered by themselves" (p. 184). The biologist no longer even asks any question as to the criterion enabling one to separate that which is hereditary and that which is secondarily adapted, but "the logician of science" (p. 185) is fortunately at hand to remind him of this question. Step by step, in thus delimiting that which is adapted from that which is inherited, then once again within the latter that which is adapted and that which is inherited, etc., we thereby arrive at the first living being. On this point, transformism and in particular Darwin remain silent. "This is perhaps a mark of scientific prudence, it is, in any case, a cause of philosophical obscurity" (p. 188).

We thus see from the first how a philosopher claiming to play the twofold rule (without, however, suspecting the intrinsic contradiction) of giving ultimate explanations and of being a logician of science, conceives the "intellectual cooperation between scientists and philosophers." Science, *ancilla philosophiae*, provides the material, and philosophy corrects the methods of elaboration, examines the interpretations, and finally prescribes its own solutions.

These solutions are in the particular case both of a disarming simplicity and of a certain richness in imprecision. Dalbiez begins by stating that finality is not a characteristic of life, but that defined as "a preordination of potentiality to the act" it occurs on the physical plane wherever there is movement or a causal relation. This is, as one knows, a belief common to Aristotelian

physics and to children up to eight or nine years of age. But at
this point Dalbiez cannot prevent himself from giving physicists
a lesson and to see "an evident vicious circle" in the assertion
of a primary statistical determinism, for "it is enough to look
carefully" in order to discover beneath it "determinism properly
so called and consequently preordination" (p. 179). The "care"
devoted by Dalbiez to this investigation has unfortunately not
prevented the great majority of nuclear physicists from taking
up the opposite position since then.

Dalbiez defines a living thing as having the characteristics of
"moving itself or acting on itself instead of acting only on
others" (p. 180), a definition leading therefore to the idea of
self-regulation, which as we know today is compatible with mechanical feedback models. In this connection Dalbiez maintains
as against most of his vitalist colleagues the possibility of spontaneous movements, *i.e.* not arising from external stimuli: the
objectivist school has, however, now proved their existence (see
Holst and others). After which comes the justification of a full-
blooded finalism: "Selection can only occur if one posits the
tendency of life to perpetuate itself" (p. 190), as if a tendency
cannot be explained by the laws of equilibrium; Lamarckian
adaptation presupposes "as soon as one reflects on it" (pp. 191–
92) "a pre-established disposition," although "as a result of
considering the modifications, one neglects the modified" (p.
192). Finally mutationism, completed appropriately by Cuénot's
"pre-adaptation," similarly involves a finalism, for despite Cuénot's clearest statements, "the theory of pre-adaptation ought
to be considered as a refined finalism" (p. 194). In other words,
if a species of mollusk that is more resistant than others to
climatic variations is accidentally transplanted to a xerothermic
region through animal fodder brought in from elsewhere, and
breeds prolifically there even at high altitudes,[6] we have here a

6 This is a real example of "pre-adaptation," that of *Xerophilia obvia*
transplanted from Eastern Europe to the Valaisian Alps, where I have followed its propagation from 1911 until today.

case of "refined finality"! Under these conditions it would be a miracle to discover events which did not exhibit finality.

Dalbiez next considers animal psychology and asserts with the same surprising dogmatism that the intelligence of animals does not exist or consists exclusively in "associative memory." The entire work of W. Köhler, whose basic study, however, appeared in 1917, flatly contradicts this interpretation.

In conclusion, according to Dalbiez transformism is a doctrine shared by two contradictory philosophies: mechanism, which denies qualities as well as time; and historicism, which leads to pure contingency. Hence the need to reconcile them by introducing finality, evidence of which may be seen from the first living being and which alone gives to a physico-chemical aggregate the property of achieving equilibrium with its environment. It brings about precisely this reconciliation of mechanism and historicism, and from the simple increase of entropy characteristic of thermodynamic equilibrium to homeostasis and self-regulations, a whole series of levels provides increasingly precise models of finality.

What this work does show is how an agrégé of philosophy, who disturbs four biologists to bring them together for the first meeting of the "Society for the Philosophy of Nature," comes, by appealing to the primacy of metaphysical knowledge, to subject them to a mixture of the commonplace and of risky or already false personal opinions. Dalbiez's only guiding method consists in "looking with care" and "reflecting on it," while modestly calling himself a "logician of science."

(D) A more serious attempt is that of R. Ruyer, who has made the effort to acquire a large amount of biological knowledge. As a prisoner of war in Germany together with the great embryologist E. Wolff, Ruyer took part in the work of the "Biology Club" of his "Oflag" in a "Prisoner of War University" directed by the great mathematician Leray. Ruyer thus found himself involved in that atmosphere of scientific interchange which is so seriously lacking in the usual training of philosophers. On returning to Nancy, Ruyer continued reading and thinking about the subject, and this led him to write, among other things, his *Eléments de psychobiologie* (P.U.F., 1946). It is therefore of some interest to see what he has derived from the synthesis of his biological knowledge and his philosophical studies.

In all justice we ought first to acknowledge a certain number of intelligent insights and of valid ideas that are to be found in this work, beginning with the project to combine into a single whole behavior and organic life; in other words, the data of psychology and that of biology. For example, Ruyer is often able to construct "true forms" (as against aggregates) in systems not coinciding with perceived wholes: *viz* that of which the adult swallow is only a segment or a subordinate cycle of the "swallow's reproductive" cycle. Ruyer thus concludes that "instinct is the aspect taken by the dynamism of the real cyclical form when it imposes itself on an individual so as to relate it to its unity" (p. 41). This of course explains nothing, but the formula is an apt one for placing the problem of instinct on a level of organization, not internal to the individual but going beyond it in space and time, and of which it is a question of abstracting the laws and structure.

But this ability to devise enlarged cycles and abstract structures for which concrete biology has a certain need, and which is beginning to be expressed in contemporary cybernetic studies (which Ruyer has followed and excellently reported on), has been insufficient to safeguard philosophy against the two great temptations which threaten all speculation in the field of life. These are the use of unverifiable explanations and the tendency to project into the elementary processes properties belonging to higher levels of behavior and of mental life.

On the first point Ruyer tells us (p. 11) that "the dynamic form behind the structure, the structuring activity, and the relationships are unobservable and ought always to be inferred at one's own risk." But from this starting point we are naturally led to ask if the valid structures we look for are not precisely those that like the important qualitative algebraic structures

contain their own laws of construction, without it being necessary to imagine "behind" them a structuring activity. In a
"group" structure, for example, the structuring activity is none
other than the operation that defines this group. If Ruyer does
not take up such an approach [7] perhaps this is because he does
not wish to see that the relationship between the functioning
of a structure and the structuring itself is to be looked for in
self-regulations or active processes of equilibrium. He distrusts
the concept of "equilibrium," as he puts it, insofar as it belongs
to physiological physico-chemistry, which is said to be a "secondary" science (p. 2) in opposition to the "primary" sciences,
or sciences of "real forms" like atomic physics, biology, and
psychology! But it is above all because Ruyer quickly leaves the
field of facts so as to proceed not only toward the moving sands
of "inferences with risk," but toward a metaphysics of the "potential." And this despite all that history teaches us respecting
the verbal manipulation of concepts that only have a meaning
in the field of precise measurement and demonstration.

In fact from pp. 12 to 15 we learn with surprise that "every
real form" presupposes a "potential" and that if the physical
potentials are to be found in space-time, the biological forms
could only occur in space and time as the actualization of a potential "trans-spatiotemporal," for, according to Cuénot, onto-
genesis is "preparatory of the future" (while we "have never
seen a heap of snow putting itself in equilibrium with a future
storm"). In other words, life is from the start presupposed as
finality (Ruyer prefers the term "thematism" to that of "finalism"—p. 187—but that comes to the same thing), and finality
justifies reference to a "potential" situated outside observable
nature. This is as much as immediately telling us that God has
arranged everything in advance and that there is no other explanation to look for.

But without being bothered by this surprising mixture of
levels, which, on the contrary, he uses as a basis for his philo-

---

[7] From which suspect formulae like: "As for instinct, since it is the
guardian of structure it could not be its resultant" (p. 42).

sophico-biological system, Ruyer nonetheless tries to find explanations of it in making a detailed use of his wealth of factual information. The manner of these explanations is then very simple: it consists in attributing to all "true forms" the characteristics of the most highly evolved forms of mental life.

For example, from p. 10 he speaks of the "subjectivity of molecules" and from p. 17 he asserts that "every force is of mental origin." As for the elementary organisms, one wants to be "particularly clear" in asserting that "the primary organic psychism is not a kind of confused and rudimentary variety of the psychism of psychology" and "is only unconscious in the precise sense of: devoid of intentional images turned toward the world," for "the psychism which guarantees and preserves the structures of an amoeba, of a plant, or of an animal is completely 'distinct.' There is nothing mysterious here, it is simply qua activity, turned 'inward' (we understand by this, toward the preservation of its own constituent elements) and not as the psychic activity of the higher animals, toward the external environment. The amoeba or the plant *erlebt, enjoys, survole*, or *thinks* . . . its organic structure with as much clarity as man thinks of the tool he is in process of making" (p. 24).

This authoritative text will not perhaps surprise every biolologist, for we know how they have often appealed to "psychoids," etc., but it will certainly surprise every psychologist concerned with effective research. Nevertheless, the consciousness of molecules seems immediately to raise two problems at least: how to establish its existence and what it could add to what we already know of these material systems? As for the psychism of the amoeba, Ruyer himself reminds us (p. 22) that the amoeba can be conditioned, acquire habits, etc., and from this he concludes that "psychism" is prior to the nervous system. After which two pages further on, this behavior evidently relative to its interaction with the environment (the amoeba "acts," says Ruyer) becomes the sign of a psychism turned only "inward" and charged with the preservation of the organic structure!

Beneath the triviality and contradictions, we only in fact

find this essentially verbal mode of explanation already noted with respect to the "potential" and which consists in assuming that by reifying a process and naming it we contribute something, whatever it might be, to the solution of the problems that it sets. The amoeba certainly exhibits "behavior," and we are acquainted with several kinds of such behavior. But do we make any advance at all in seeing therein the expression of a "psychism"? Psychism, if we must use this term, is just the set of behavioral activities and not at all their cause. To say that the amoeba "thinks" with the same clarity as a man making a tool, is either word-spinning or a way of saying that its behavior forms an initial stage of that which will become intelligence. In the latter case we have simply stated a problem of structural analysis and of relationship, but strictly speaking we say nothing more in speaking already at this stage of thought and intelligence, for these are words empty of meaning as long as we have not described and interpreted each of the mechanisms occurring at the levels of the development considered. The psychism brought in by Ruyer is therefore completely devoid of meaning for a psychologist: it is only the statement of a problem, and a bad statement into the bargain.

But there is worse to come. In assuming from the start that this kind of soul attributed to the amoeba explains everything in the constitution or maintenance of its organic structure, we obscure important problems. Those raised on the one hand, by the hypothesis that the mechanism of this structuring is at the same time the cause of the corresponding behavior, or on the other, by the hypothesis that there are two kinds of organization that are complementary or which interact. We have here a group of problems as fundamental for psychology as for biology, and one is surprised that a writer so well informed can thus settle, by means of sweeping statements completely devoid of verification, what will require decades or centuries of research.

This criticism may seem severe. But we merely need to read the way in which Ruyer deals with the very honest L. Bertalanffy, whose work has an entirely different scientific basis and a depth with which the author cannot compare: "The conceptions of Bertalanffy lack clarity. They perfectly represent a shamefaced vitalism and consequently a confused one" (p. 193, n.l). If Bertalanffy is a confused vitalist what shall we say of R. Ruyer?

For the latter, the whole of biology is explained by consciousness, and this simply because it is a "flexible and patterning force, which exhibits itself in a primary fashion in the patterning of organic forms . . . , etc." (p. 293). But consciousness is at the same time "apperception of essences and values." And it is by this even the origin of memory: "The status of mnemonic entities is quite similar to that of essences and values. The mnemonic entities are beyond existents. Memory is beyond the spatio-temporal plane" (p. 293). This is then the result of biological mentalism: memory is beyond time (oh Bergson!), life is beyond nature . . . and truth is beyond all verification.

(E) If we pass from biology to psychology, we find that the interventions of philosophers in questions of fact, properly so called, naturally increase, and even to the nth power. The first reason for this is the lacunary character of this still young science, which is even now only in its early stages. P. Fraisse ends his chapter on "The Evolution of Experimental Psychology," in the _Traité_, which we published together, as follows: "The territory which it has conquered is increasingly large, but the ground has scarcely been cleared. The modern history of psychology is only beginning" (Part I, p. 69). It follows that the as yet unexplored regions leave the field open to speculation, and a very much wider one than in biology. The second reason is that even in questions in which research has been in progress for a number of years, the philosopher has assumed that he had the right to consider and actively discuss such questions from the sole fact that the phenomena concerned dealt with the internal world. It is not for nothing that a philosopher of common sense like Dalbiez limits science, in one of the quoted passages (under B), to knowledge of the external world. Internal phenomena have the advantage of an established tradition and the criticisms directed to the methods of introspection in no way prevent philosophical common sense from postulating implicitly or explicitly that in such a domain "reflection" remains supreme.

Let us therefore try to see what this leads to in questions of fact. We shall not return to the discussion of the conflict between philosophical and scientific psychology, with which Chapter Four has been concerned. Instead we shall give several examples of the way in which philosophers have concerned themselves with questions in the field of scientific psychology itself.

The number of examples we could give here would be very large and we need to limit them. As this little work is from beginning to end a defense of scientific method in the study of mental phenomena, I will therefore restrict my examples to the reaction of French-speaking Swiss philosophers [8] to our Geneva studies in genetic psychology and epistemology.

In this respect a preliminary remark can be made that is of some interest. The *Société romande de Philosophie* was founded about forty years ago by a group of philosophers, mathematicians, logicians, psychologists ("*Je pense, donc j'en suis,*" had replied Larguier de Bancels to show that he was a member of it), linguists, etc. Its chief interest being the philosophy of science, there was no conflict then between epistemological studies, particularly historico-critical ones, and psychological studies. With the decline of epistemological interests and the collaboration of mathematicians, the new generation of philosophers accepting more specific metaphysical positions showed itself increasingly reserved with respect to genetic considerations, as if they found the latter suspect.

For example, J. B. Grize has read a paper to the *Société romande de Philosophie* on *Logique et psychologie de l'intelligence* in which, in his function as a logician collaborating with the psychologists of our center, he was in a good position to show the epistemological significance of psychogenesis without contradicting logic. But the philosopher D. Christoff has argued

[8] I.e., those of the *Suisse Romande* (Trs.).

that the question how the subject has acquired an insight into something as self-evident "is not of the same order [as the latter] and changes nothing as far as the nature of self-evidence is concerned." [9] We all know, however, that even in mathematics (and Fiala reminded him of this shortly afterward in connection with the principle of excluded middle), the concept of self-evidence changes throughout history, and sometimes as a result of sudden intellectual crises. How can we therefore refuse to acknowledge that the way in which a self-evident judgment is formed can elucidate its soundness or weakness according to whether, for example, it is related to the very general coordinations of actions and operations, or whether it depends, like certain out-of-date self-evident judgments of geometry, on limiting factors of perception or imagery rather than on these constant operational coordinations?

R. Schaerer shifted the question on to the field of moral judgments and referred to my work on their evolution. "There is a directed passage,[10] Piaget tells us, from heteronomy to autonomy, from egocentricism to reciprocity and to solidarity. The philosopher asks him; (1) to justify this directed passage, which appears to be in contradiction with the revisability of principles and the unpredictable character of future events . . . ; (2) to avoid the use of terms loaded with ethical meaning such as 'autonomy,' 'reciprocity,' and 'solidarity' " (p. 247). The charm of this language will be immediately appreciated: "The philosopher asks him to justify . . . and to avoid . . .", which closely echoes that of R. Dalbiez, who offered his advice to the biologists (see Chapter Two). Here are my answers.

On the first point there is a contradiction between R. Schaerer and H. Mieville, whom, however, he calls in to the rescue. On the field of the rational norms of the subject, Mieville (see Chapter One under D) had tried to oppose the notions of revisability and unpredictability by accepting the directed

---

[9] *Revue de philosophie et de théologie*, Lausanne, 1962, p. 245.
[10] I use the phrase "directed passage" for Piaget's technical term *vection* (Trs.).

passage I have described, but maintaining that it implies the absolute norm, which I claimed to do without. This very consistent position has not convinced me, for the existence of a directed passage can be verified without projecting on to it the observer's mental norms, and without the latter referring to an absolute (revisable norms suffice as long as there is not a necessary revision). Schaerer, on the other hand, wanted at first to show there was a contradiction between the verification of a directed passage and the principle of revisability, which is meaningless, since a verification is always revisable and a directed passage can only cover a partial period of development, and undergoes later changes that are effectively unpredictable as long as they remain unverified. In wanting me to "justify" my assertions he forgets that the task of the experimenter is to proceed cautiously before asserting the existence of a fact, and that these safeguards have been adequate, for similar results have been found by investigators in the U.S.A., at Louvain, Montreal, etc., and in very different environments. Schaerer's demands are therefore particularly surprising here. It is, on the contrary, for the psychologist to ask him to justify his concern with questions of fact unless, of course, he may have taken the phrase "directed passage" in a different sense and not understood that it is a question of a simple law of development, although concerning the evolution of norms that the subjects recognize or take as given.

On the second point, Schaerer wants to correct my terminology and advises me to use "axiologically" neutral terms. I will be bold enough to resist this, since my problem is that of the evolution of the norms of the subjects which I study, without concerning myself with my own nor those of the philosopher Schaerer. The value of the terms "autonomy" and "reciprocity" is that they allow us to study the possible parallelism between the development of moral norms and intellectual norms without confusing them. But the question is, of course, not about these verbal disputes. It depends on the fact that for philosophers like R. Schaerer the psychological study of the evolution of the norms of the subject that develop gradually between childhood and adult age, has not the least interest as far as our knowledge of the adult mind is concerned. In other words, psychogenetic analysis is only a pure and simple description and has no explanatory value. It is on this central point that it would seem useful to continue the discussion.

Schaerer returned to this question at the 1962 *Rencontres internationales de Genève* in unambiguous terms: "M. Piaget's conclusions extended into the domain . . . of philosophy, become singularly questionable and . . . one might even say that it produces a certain reversal of positions" (*La vie et le temps*, p. 205). Let us therefore see what this reversal is worth. Schaerer takes up again the directed passage from egocentricism to autonomy and reciprocity, but this time he says of it: "This conclusion extended on to the philosophical plane, can become singularly dangerous" (p. 205). The proof of it is (and this "philosophical" extension will be admired) the following little story. Let us suppose, says the philosopher, that I have been involved in sharp practices and that a shady lawyer has successfully defended me, while my little child seeing me upset throws himself into my arms to comfort me. In this case: "Where is the reciprocity and the solidarity? From the instrumental point of view, from the operational point of view which is, I believe, that of M. Piaget, it is with the dishonest lawyer. He alone has been able to put himself in my place and to get me out of trouble. The child is completely unable to do this" (p. 206). And then "the reversal to which I have just referred takes place," the philosopher concludes: in reality it is "the child who is better than we are!"

I would like to point out three small difficulties. The first is the confusion of the subjects' intellectual and moral norms, whose parallelism I have tried to show, but not their identity. The lawyer of the story is intelligent, but cannot serve as an example for moral norms. I have therefore answered Schaerer that I do not see here any moral reciprocity nor solidarity, but at the most complicity (moral reciprocity is recognized as a necessary conservation of values and is completely lacking here). And as the philosopher persisted, I asked him to define his terms. But

Schaerer replied, "As Pascal has said, to wish to define certain terms which speak for themselves is to obscure the question." We are therefore put into the picture. . . .

The second ambiguity concerns the hierarchy of norms and their application. To say that the child is more moral than the adult can be understood in two completely different senses, according to whether the question is "How do subjects evaluate norms?" [11] or "To what extent (from the point of view of fact or sincerity, etc.) do they apply them?" Let us suppose that all (or almost all) subjects of a certain level (of age, etc.) consider norms B as superior to norms A, for example, reciprocity in relation to obedience, or the morality of the New Testament in relation to a legalistic morality. I will speak in this case of a directed passage from A to B, but it can well be that norms B, precisely because they are superior, are less well applied. Schaerer's expression "the child is better than we are" is therefore without meaning as long as one has not specified whether "better" refers to the level of norms or to the way in which they are observed. If we agree that the child is "better" from this second point of view (subject to verification), this proves nothing as far as the question under discussion is concerned.

The third difficulty concerns the concepts of equilibrium and reversibility in which R. Schaerer sees only instrumental processes without relation to logical or moral norms, in denying, moreover, that equilibrium is compatible with development, and reversibility with irreversible decisions. But here again I will ask for a discussion with definitions and formal demonstrations. It goes without saying that if we speak of equilibrium in the ordinary sense of a balance of opposing forces, Schaerer would be right. but he needs to understand that a biological equilibrium is self-regulating, and that self-regulatory systems provide mechanical models of finality, and he ought also to learn something about the logistic analysis of decision-making, which does not at all exclude the use of reversible operations. He would then

[11] Or to put it more clearly, "Which norms do they accept?" or "What level do their norms belong to (in a possible hierarchy)?"

better understand that the changing equilibrium of systems of concepts or values can characterize cognitive mechanisms as well as those of the will, and that it has for the subject a normative meaning and not only an instrumental one.

If I stress these endless discussions with R. Schaerer, it is because they raise a general problem of methodology. We have to explain how a professor of the history of philosophy can discuss questions of fact, which have been subjected for some years now and in several countries to detailed experimental verification, remaining satisfied with commonsense arguments, verbal approximations of a most summary kind, and such distressing examples as the little story of the dishonest lawyer and the affectionate child.

There is only one explanation for this: the belief that a competency in questions of norms involves by that very fact, knowledge of the mechanisms of the subject's conduct. The moral philosopher discusses values or norms as such, and they do not, of course, concern the psychologist. But in studying individual subjects, the latter verifies that they take as given or recognize norms, whence a series of problems. What are the norms of subjects? Are they constant or do they evolve with age? By what processes does the subject come to feel that he is bound by them? Are these processes the same at every age or do they change? etc. These are questions of fact, "normative facts," *i.e.* norms for the subject and facts for the observer, but pure facts for the latter, since he neither prescribes nor evaluates anything as far as these subjective norms are concerned. If Schaerer feels obliged to concern himself with these questions, and even to stipulate that I used a different terminology, it is because he believes that his competency with regard to norms gives him knowledge of what is going on in the subjects' minds. These are two entirely distinct questions, so different that in the parallel normative domain of logic, for more than half a century logicians have realized that their analyses of truth involved no knowledge of the way in which subjects actually reasoned. And these remarks, of course, apply equally well to the adult as well as to the child.

The philosopher will say that he knows himself. This remains to be seen, for as we have observed in Chapter Four, an introspection verified by reference to several people is one thing, and an introspection restricted to a self who is both judge and party and who as subject imposes his philosophy on the self-object attended to, is quite another. But even to know oneself at a time *t* does not give any knowledge of the earlier formative and developmental stages of which the adult mind is at least the partial resultant. To understand this development, which alone has an explanatory power, it is no longer consciousness itself which has to be examined, but the whole of conduct of which consciousness is a function and only one function. Conduct presupposes an analysis of facts with well-tried methods that alone allow objectivity to be attained, not in the sense of neglecting the subject, but in the sense of correcting the distortions due to the observer's self. An historian of Greek thought ought to be the first to understand that ideas rarely have an absolute beginning and that the relationships between ideas cannot be reconstructed by reflection alone or by fictitious examples.

(F) An instructive object lesson, as far as these misunderstandings are concerned, is F. L. Mueller's *Histoire de la psychologie de l'Antiquité à nos jours*, which was followed by a small book on *La psychologie contemporaine*, which reproduces part of the former and completes it in some respects. Mueller has definite opinions and wishes to defend philosophical psychology, while trying to remain objective with respect to scientific psychology. But as he does not believe in the latter, and since a philosopher's education consists in studying texts and not the different methods by which knowledge is increased, he has studied extremely conscientiously the writings of psychologists. However, he has not realized that in order to appreciate what is being done in scientific psychology, he ought to have undertaken some effective research on some topic that is breaking new ground. This would have been closer to that living and humane understanding which he constantly opposes to intellectualism. It is therefore of some interest to see how a philosopher who does not belong to any philosophical school judges scientific psychology.

In a general fashion, it is surprising that a historian of ideas should not have known better how to separate the important tendencies in the history of psychology, tendencies naturally connected (by action and reaction) to the evolution of methods. Starting mainly from physiological psychology and psychophysics, with especial emphasis on the methods of generalized measurement, then using the method of tests, scientific psychology has later been enriched by psycho-pathological studies. From this, on the one hand, has emerged psychoanalysis, and on the other, two great movements, in France and in Great Britain, the latter more physiological and the former, with Janet, soon interesting itself in a general psychology of conduct and also a genetic psychology, on this latter point, moreover, resembling psychoanalysis itself. The earlier physiological psychology having given rise to a much too empiricist and mechanist doctrine, namely associationism, a reaction occurred from the end of the last century and the beginning of the twentieth in the form of American functionalism [12] (from the time of James), and the fundamental verifications introduced by the method of controlled introspection (Binet and the Würzburg school), which has invalidated the explanation of intelligence by means of association and images. The initial method of these later studies was too restricted and the functionalist tendency has thus produced, as in psycho-pathology, an increasingly general point of view in psychology which is the study of conduct in general including consciousness; Watson's behaviorism being an extreme example and under this form only temporary. On the other hand, laboratory psychology, whose activities have not been curtailed by these many complementary studies, has been given a new lease of life by Gestalt theory, which, moreover, has also become concerned with the study of conduct in general, while the latter

[12] And that of Claparède from 1903 (*L'association des idées*).

has become differentiated into genetic psychology, social psychology, etc.

F. L. Mueller's two books do not exhibit these different streams of thought in their interconnections and significance, nor especially in their deeper convergences. A philosopher, in fact, is interested more in the differences of schools and systems, and experiences in his field a somewhat professional pleasure when theories arise showing a marked divergence from the existing ones. Thus the most important chapter of the *Histoire* concerned with the "new" psychology called "The schools and fields of inquiry," becomes in the second volume "The methods and fields of inquiry," but without any more emphasis on the relationship between these methods. A psychologist, on the other hand, is much more concerned with the unity of psychology and the increasing convergence of his methods.

Let us take psychoanalysis as an example. Mueller points out that "exact scientists go so far as to deny any scientific character to it" (I, p. 385; II, p. 56). The exact scientist quoted in support of this statement is none other than Marcel Boll, who knows logic and many other things but who has never done anything in psychology except, as all amateurs do, some characterology (and who has pilloried not only the psychoanalysts but many other thinkers in different fields of inquiry).

But if psychoanalysis is the only field of psychology in which one can effectively speak of "schools," it is because the Freudians, etc., have wanted for professional reasons to form closed groups in order to safeguard the practice of their techniques. The difficulty is that as everywhere where there is a "school" its members convince themselves too easily and therefore develop too few of the habits of verification, and it is solely for this reason that experimentalists experience misgivings in connection with certain facts and interpretations still unverified. The best proof that it is a question of a legitimate attitude is that several Freudians have for some years now been concerned with experimental verification, and with a more general restructuring of the theory. This is particularly the case with the group formed at

Stockbridge under the stimulus of the late D. Rapaport (Wolff, Erikson, etc.).[13] And if we want an example of the attitude of someone who passes as a critic of the Freudian interpretation in 1920 I gave a lecture to the *Société Alfred Binet* in Paris on the psychoanalytical movement, which was printed in the *Bulletin* of that Society at a time when, as Mueller recalls, this subject was little discussed in France. At the same time I underwent a didactic psychoanalysis in order to understand something about it, and in 1922 I read a paper on *La pensée de l'enfant*, with Freud being present, at the Psycho-analytical Congress in Berlin. Again, the School of Psychiatry at Topeka (Kansas), known as the Mecca of American Freudianism, invited me several years ago to stay some weeks there so as to discuss common problems. One thus sees that the existence of schools does not in psychology exclude the search for convergences, nor above all the verification of facts giving a meaning to this inquiry.

To return to the main tendencies of contemporary scientific psychology, two lacunae are striking in Mueller's works. The first is that little attempt has been made to isolate the most general of these tendencies, which is to establish a psychology of "conduct," including consciousness, but relating it to the whole of behavior, external or internalized. The latter is not at all neglected despite Watson, who had, moreover, retained "internal speech," which he had strongly stressed. In this respect, it is very significant to see how little Mueller has understood the work of P. Janet (whom he often quotes, however) and particularly its evolution: the passage from a static theory based on the idea of synthesis and of automatism to a conception of the hierarchy of functions and from there to a theory of stages at once genetic and psycho-pathological, including fixations and disinte-

---

[13] From these investigations and from those which they have influenced, two books have appeared, among others, showing the convergence between the psychoanalytical data concerning the first two years of life and my analyses of the same sensori-motor levels: Wolff, *The developmental psychologies of Jean Piaget and Psycho-analysis.* Psych. Issues, 1960, and T. Gouin-Décarie, *Intelligence et affectivité chez le jeune enfant,* Delachaux et Niestlé.

grations. The most important part of this work, where influence will be permanent, is the interpretation of affectivity as a regulation of action together with the detailed table of regulations of activation and termination corresponding to the "elementary sentiments" of which Janet gave the most perceptive description. It is difficult to see how he can overlook all this in order to conclude at the end of the book that the objectivism of scientific psychology makes it miss the problem of the subject. To understand this phenomenon one needs to refer to the varied reasons for this lack of understanding which I have tried to describe in this little work.

But there is more to it. We look with interest at how Mueller tries to reconcile these theses on "objectivism" with the studies carried out from the beginning of this century on controlled introspection, a method discovered and used by the German psychologists of the Würzburg school and by Binet in Paris. The reconciliation is very simple. Mueller tells us nothing about this important occurrence, and the names of Kulpe, Marbe, and of the great K. Bühler, are not to be found in the table of contents. Of Binet's book on this subject, published in 1903, we only find the following mention, the skillfulness of which will be appreciated. Binet "indicates the difference between his approach and that of laboratory psychology. Experimentation as he conceived it is therefore very extensive. It specifically includes questionnaires, interviews, experimental investigations, etc., that is to say procedures which involve the use of controlled introspection" (p. 387). This is just as if Binet and the Würzburg school had not wanted explicitly to use controlled introspection in order to exploit it to the full. It is only a question of the discovery of a method to be sure, since after several years it has resulted in something else, but it is important because it has specifically led to many other things. The Würzburg school, after having given acute analyses that demonstrated the independence of judgment in relation to association and the image, has been unable to elucidate the mechanism of this judgment by introspection alone. Later investigators have had to proceed to more functional and above all extrospective studies, like Selz and Lindworski for thought in general, and Claparède for the origin of the hypothesis (with his method of "spoken reflection," which certainly concentrates on the subject, but not merely by introspection alone). As for Binet, if the use of the same method of controlled introspection has cured him of associationism, he has seen from the start that it deals with resultants of thought and not its mechanisms, and has concluded with the well-known paradox, "Thought is an unconscious activity of the mind" in order to proceed to study the psychology of conduct.

If Mueller thus surprisingly omits certain important trends of psychological thought, those which he includes equally need commenting on as far as his actual understanding of them is concerned. Mueller feels, for example, sympathy for Gestalt psychology because it has been influenced by phenomenology. However, one knows that this is only in the sense that in both cases there is an interaction between subject and object. He specifically asks if the famous experiments of Köhler on chimpanzees have not been biased by the influence of imitation. This is evidence of a worthy interest on his part in the isolation of experimental factors but it also shows that he has read little of Köhler, for the latter has taken care to verify, among other things, that contrary to the usual view, the ape does not "ape" and only imitates that which he understands. On the other hand, Mueller has understood neither the purpose nor even the meaning of Köhler's theory of "physical forms" (soap bubbles, surface of water, etc.). Its purpose was to explain the perceptual or other "good forms" by the laws of equilibrium of the field, in accordance with the hypothesis that there is an isomorphism between the "forms" of consciousness and the organization of the electrical fields occurring in the nervous sytesm. W. Köhler, who was a physicist before being a psychologist (as Wallach was a chemist), then tried to show that the structure of the Gestalt defined by its nonadditive composition (action of the whole on the parts without the whole being equivalent to their sum) is found in the physical world, but together with structures involving additive compositions. A mechanical summation like the parallelogram of forces is therefore not a Gestalt, while one finds Gestalten in the laws of field equilibrium (where we need to note that the compositions are irreversible because they are partly due to chance). Failing to understand them, Mueller regards these bold but plausible hypotheses as metaphysical in character (which is what positivist opponents of Gestalt theory have perhaps said) and as setting a "philosophical problem" (II, p. 93). We can certainly find philosophical problems everywhere, but it would be interesting to know what the ideas of the philosopher Mueller could add to those of the physicist and psychologist Köhler. I am not saying this in order to defend the Gestalt thesis. On the contrary, all that I accept of Köhler's analysis is that just as the physical universe exhibits reversible phenomena (mechanical) and irreversible ones (thermodynamical, etc.), mental life similarly exhibits irreversible structures (Gestalten) and reversible ones (operational intelligence), the latter therefore being irreducible to the former. But I cannot at all see by what criterion a writer who has so quickly understood Köhler's main theses can say to him: look out, or you will see that you are philosophizing!

As for Mueller's very friendly and careful account of my own work, which is full of sympathetic understanding, I readily agree, on the other hand, that my studies raise philosophical problems, since their aim has been to test by psychogenetic experiment a certain number of hypotheses as to the growth of knowledge, and these hypotheses can be generalized or discussed within the field of epistemology. But on two or three points I have had difficulty in following Mueller.

The first is his assertion according to which the progressive equilibrium of the cognitive mechanisms from childhood to adult age would simply be the description of the "goal" followed and not an explanation (pp. 423–24). To begin with, the concept of equilibrium specifically allows us to get away from that of finality. I have then tried to show (*Logique et équilibre,*

P.U.F., 1956) that the process of equilibrium is based on a succession of increasing sequential probabilities, such that each stage *becomes* the most probable, after the occurrence of the preceding one without being it from the start, which is a probabilist explanation, true or false but plausible. Finally, equilibrium leads to operational reversibility and results from increasingly complex systems of regulations whose roots are to be looked for in the most fundamental organic processes, which at the very least form a sufficiently wide explanatory perspective.

In the second place, Mueller says that I claim "not to leave the ground of experience itself" and adds "but the question is whether he is really successful and what price he pays for this" (p. 424). Let me first remark that if one states what this price is, as Mueller does in saying that I only arrive at "a form of empty universality, purely scientific" (p. 426), this means that I do not leave the ground of experience. But if I really understand his logic, which is neither "empty" nor therefore "scientific," I am unsuccessful in this while paying the same price as if I had been successful.

Let us reply to the first question, which is ambiguous, however, without a definition of "experience." If it is that of empiricism I certainly do not accept it, being anti-empiricist. If we are concerned with scientific experience it always involves a question, an answer given by the facts, and an interpretation. The question is an open one, provided that it can be so put that it can be answered by the facts. As for the interpretation, it consists in explanatory hypotheses that give rise to new questions, which in turn provide direct or indirect verification for these hypotheses in accordance with the deductions made from them, and these new questions require new factual answers and new interpretations, etc. Thought of in this way, experience is therefore inseparable from deductive inferences, which will be considered as valid if they are formalized, or if without being so they agree intuitively with logical or mathematical models. To say or suggest as Mueller does, that I go beyond the field of experience can therefore have two meanings; either that I state problems that cannot be answered by the facts (or to which they do not give an answer) or that I interpret these answers in non-verifiable terms (either that the explanatory hypotheses are no longer verifiable by other facts, or that they involve logical inconsistencies). All this is possible, and I therefore hope that F. L. Mueller will amplify his remarks. But if he wishes merely to say, as one might suspect from his remarks on Köhler, that while believing that I concern myself with experience I am really philosophizing, my reply would be that according to the preceding definition of experience, which seems to me to be a common one, to philosophize would mean to assert nonverifiable or nonlogical propositions, and this is not a very fruitful conception. In a general fashion I will also ask him in the name of what criteria and by what right does the philosopher intervene in the work of the experimenter, in order to tell him whether or not he goes beyond experience, and whether he believes he is justified in doing this only with respect to the psychologist or whether he would also include the biologist and the physicist.

Moreover, Mueller's purpose is clear from the context of pp. 424–25: he would like me to say that my psychology is closely bound up with the Marxist dialectic, as Wallon, rightly or wrongly, has said of his own. And further he would like me, in terms of this dialectic, to distinguish more clearly between psychology and genetic epistemology, as was suggested to me by the philosopher Kedrov after a somewhat subjective or tendentious report of R. Zazzo [14] quoted by Mueller during a discussion we

---

[14] Zazzo's report only incompletely reproduces the beginning of the discussion, which I have summarized in the *American Psychologist* after having had my text checked by one of the principal Soviet psychologists in order to avoid errors of interpretation. I did not first raise the problem of idealism, but the philosopher Kedrov opened the discussion by asking me the question "Do you believe that the object exists before knowledge?" I replied: "As a psychologist I know nothing of this, for I only know the object in acting on it and I can say nothing about it before this action." Rubinstein then proposed the conciliatory formula: "For us the object is a part of the world. Do you believe that the world exists before knowledge?" I then said (and not with reference to the subject): "This is another matter. In order to act on the object it is necessary for there to be an organism

had at the Moscow Academy of Sciences. If there are definite points of convergence between my interpretations and the dialectic, as L. Goldmann, M. Rubel, C. Nowinski, and others have noted, I would like to make it clear that it is a matter of convergence and not of influence (even at second-hand, as M. Rubel deplores it) and that it is better for the two sides. As we have seen in Chapter Three (under F), either the dialectic is a metaphysics like any other, which claims to direct science, and this can only harm science as well as itself, or its strength is due to the fact that it converges with all manner of spontaneous scientific ideas, and the only thing to do therefore is to work in complete independence.

One last point: the price of my position "imbued with logic and epistemology" (p. 421) is therefore to end in "an empty universality, purely scientific" (p. 426), and unable to provide a "philosophical anthropology." The whole of this book is my answer to remarks of this kind, so often heard. But these remarks are, on the other hand, the best justification for the need for such a work. All that a twentieth-century philosopher who has read Sartre and Merleau-Ponty but written a "history of psychology" without having practiced it, finds to say of this scientific ideal is that it consists of an empty "universality." Because living philosophy, that of Plato, Aristotle, Descartes, Leibniz, or Kant, has given rise to a series of disciplines that have become independent, a twentieth-century philosopher, if he is neither a logician,

---

and this organism is also part of the world. I therefore evidently believe that the world exists before all knowledge, but that we only divide it up into individual objects through our actions and as a result of an interaction between the organism and the environment." At this moment a discussion in Russian occurred, at the end of which I facetiously said, "I have not entirely understood, but I have, however, grasped two words: 'Piaget' and 'idealism.' Might I ask their connection?" It is at this point (and not after the reflections on psychology and epistemology as Zazzo has said, with the reservation made by him) that in substance Rubinstein has stated: "We have decided that Piaget is not an idealist." After which the conversation turned to the relationships between psychology and epistemology and Kedrov made the profound remark: "You tend to psychologize epistemology and we to epistemologize psychology."

nor an epistemologist, nor a psychologist, only finds a *raison d'être* by opposing a "philosophical anthropology" to what for him is an empty universality. One may ask what its content will be.[15] Bergsonism? Mueller has noted the inadequacy of the "innermost self" alien to all action. Phenomenology? Mueller has seen the basic difficulty involved in the latter's assumption of an absolute beginning of experience completely independent of history. The dialectic? But practitioners of the Marxist dialectic in Eastern Europe in no way despise scientific development, and they have certainly not thought of constructing a philosophical psychology on the fringe of scientific psychology, which is much to their credit. Then what?

The answer seems to be given in the conclusion of the "History," but in fact this conclusion is based on two ambiguities. In the first place Mueller concludes that there would not be any break between the "old" and the "new" psychology. These expressions have certainly been used by many others and for varied ends. But from the point of view of history, which is that of the author, not two but three movements are to be distinguished, one initial and the two others contemporary but occurring later than the first.

The initial movement antedates an autonomous scientific psychology and also, which is instructive, the philosophical parascientific tendency originating in the twentieth century. We are concerned with a psychology more or less occasional or systematic according to the circumstances, elaborated by philosophers themselves, but at a time when their respective philosophies were both a reflection on science and matrices for developing sciences. For this part of his work, which extends from the

[15] Mueller therefore regards my work as useless for a "philosophical anthropology." This is not the opinion of all philosophers. See, for example, M. de Mey's article (*Anthropologie philosophique et psychologie génétique, Studia philosophica Gandensia,* 1964, pp. 41–67), which concludes that my psychology "can make a real contribution to philosophical anthropology" (p. 67). See also C. G. Granger's article (*Jean Piaget et la psychologie génétique, Critique,* 1965, pp. 249–61), which calls me a scientific humanist and believes it can discover relationships between phenomenology and my investigations.

Greeks to the eighteenth century, Mueller's analyses are excellent. He stresses the value of the philosopher's studies as much as he later tempers his evaluation of scientific psychology; he gives a very broad perspective of what has been done and above all seen by a large number of thinkers. But is this "philosophical psychology" in the twentieth-century sense, and what would Aristotle, Descartes, or Kant have said if they had to take sides in a debate comparable to that occurring today? It is clear, on the contrary, that psychology before the present schism was both scientific and philosophical insofar as it tried to grasp the facts, but introducing in different degrees factors depending on the whole of the system. The term "older" psychology is therefore essentially ambiguous.

As for the two contemporary psychologies, which we have labeled scientific and philosophical respectively, we have seen that the "break" applies only to the methods, hence to the delimitation of problems and to the mode of verification, but not to the problems themselves. If the International Union of Scientific Psychology, which nevertheless represents a general point of view, has consistently refused to be part of the International Council of Philosophy and the Human Sciences, it is certainly not because its members are disinterested in man in all his aspects, it is only because of the need to distinguish the methods used. And if we refer to it once again, it is because Mueller's writings are a fresh example of this dialogue of the deaf between two sorts of thinkers whose positions could be summarized as follows: "You wish to be objective, therefore you neglect the subject" and "You only see the universal subject through your self."

In this lies the second ambiguity of Mueller's conclusions. It is worthwhile quoting from them the central passage: "Today as yesterday, the fundamental question: what is man? remains. And in principle it excludes any answer on the field alone of the biological and psychological sciences. For it is not a question of man as a product of nature, as one object among all those which our universe contains, but of man as subject" (p. 428). In other words, scientific psychology does not study the subject, and the subject does not form part of nature; such are the two conclusions of a *Histoire de la psychologie*. If it is a question of belief in transcendent realities and of the position of man in relation to this absolute, we can only respect such points of view, but it is a question then of the problem of the coordination of values, not of pure knowledge. On the other hand, if it is a question of knowing what the subject is in relation to nature, and it seems that it is this of which Mueller speaks, then let us distinguish. To say: biology has not yet understood the nature of life and here is the enormous list of questions still outstanding of such a kind that in proportion to their solution, if it is ever completely achieved, the meaning of the term "nature" will be profoundly changed; and scientific psychology has not yet exhausted the analysis of the subject and here are the many questions that one could not pass an opinion on, etc. This would be to make a useful and constructive criticism, in which the philosopher could play his part in helping to clarify these problems. But to assert arrogantly that the question of the human "subject" excludes in principle every scientific answer is simply to include oneself in the long line of prophets, who have throughout time and in all fields fixed limits or foretold failures to the greater merit of those who have finally contradicted their prophecies. This would be unimportant if these prophecies were only negative. But they also in general offer a solution. "Man cannot live on trust alone," as Ortega y Gasset, who is quoted by F. L. Mueller, says. It then follows that for every unsolved question, one will remain dissatisfied by a position of wisdom, "provisional morality," "bets" or postulates of practical reason, but will put forward suprascientific modes of knowledge whose variety certainly proves their richness, if we are each satisfied with our personal position, a richness that is a sign of poverty if one takes as a mark of knowledge not objectivity itself but simply consistency and noncontradiction. F. L. Mueller has not observed the "com-

P

mon denominator" among the varied tendencies of scientific psychology, because he has not perhaps looked for them long enough. I would like him to point out those he observes among the different philosophical conceptions of the "human" subject.

Conclusion

"MAN CANNOT do without philosophy," says Jaspers rightly. "Moreover, it is always and everywhere present. . . . The only question which arises is to know if it is conscious or not, good or bad, confused or clear." [1] Indeed, the search for scientific truth, which, however, only interests a minority of thinkers, does not at all exhaust the nature of man, even in this minority. Man also lives, takes sides, believes in a multiplicity of values, orders them hierarchically and thus gives a meaning to his existence by decisions that constantly go beyond the limits of his actual knowledge. In the thinking man this coordination can only be a rational one, in the sense that in order to produce a synthesis between that which he believes and that which he knows he can only use reflection, either extending his knowledge or examining it critically in an effort to determine its present boundaries and to justify the acceptance of values that go beyond it. This rational synthesis between beliefs, whatever they be, and the conditions of knowledge is what we have called a "wisdom," and this seems to us to be the object of philosophy.

The term "wisdom" has nothing intellectualist about it, since it implies the taking up of a vital position. Nor has it a limiting character from the point of view of actual thinking, since it requires that this position be a rational and not an arbi-

[1] K. Jaspers, *Introduction à la philosophie*, translation, J. Hersch, Plon, pp. 7–8.

trary one. But if a wisdom includes the search for truth it must distinguish, if it is prudent, between the taking up of personal positions and those of restricted groups, relative to beliefs that are self-evident for some but not shared by others, and demonstrable truths open to everyone. In other words, there can be several wisdoms, while there exists only one truth.

The aim of this book has only been to stress this distinction. And the proof that there is nothing discreditable about it from the point of view of a professional contemporary philosopher, is that a thinker as listened to as Jaspers makes it explicitly: "The essence of philosophy is the search for truth *and not its possession* [our italics], even if as often happens it betrays itself by degenerating into knowledge stated in a set form . . . to philosophize is *to be on one's way*" (p. 8). It is these self-betrayals of philosophy that we have constantly questioned, and not philosophy as such.

From these premises Jaspers draws the following conclusions, which are precisely ours: "In philosophy there is no consensus of opinion, establishing a definitive knowledge. . . . Contrary to science, philosophy under all its forms ought to dispense with a consensus of opinion, this ought to be implicit in its very nature" (p. 2). This "philosophy without science" (p. 3; *i.e.* without knowledge) is that which we call a wisdom, and Jaspers goes so far as to derive from it the main conclusion which has been the subject of Chapters Two to Four: "*As soon as knowledge is imposed upon each individual for apoditic reasons, it becomes immediately scientific, it ceases to be philosophy and belongs to a particular domain of the knowable*" (p. 2, our italics). Without changing a single word, this is what we have tried to show from the point of view of the progressive differentiation of historical philosophies into particular scientific disciplines.

It is a natural phenomenon that philosophers, for many reasons that we have tried to analyze and which depend on the psycho-sociological motives of this social or professional class they have been able to form, constantly forget such principles of wisdom and believe they are in process of attaining a set of "particular" truths (in the sense of the last passage quoted from Jaspers). In itself this is innocuous, since each new generation forgets this Penelope's task of previous generations. It is certainly not against such tendencies that a psychologist would need to revolt, and it would be presumptuous for him to do so.

But the serious situation against which we must strongly protest, is that this tendency to establish philosophical "truths," these "pretensions, mutually exclusive, to truth," as Jaspers further says (p. 13), is accompanied today in several Western schools of philosophy by a systematically reactionary and often aggressive spirit with respect to young sciences, which limit themselves to their own studies. What was only illusion as far as the intention of completing the lacunae of science by metaphysics was concerned, becomes then error and sometimes deception. It is on this ground, where intellectual honesty is finally concerned, that it is important in certain cases to recall, limiting oneself moreover to rehabilitating the positions of the great philosophers of the past, that if philosophers wish their subject to be a general coordination of values, there exist values of objectivity and painstaking verification with which their studies have not given them close acquaintance and which they ought not as such neglect.

It is perfectly legitimate for the philosopher to feel the need to concern himself with the limits of science, but on two conditions: not to overlook those of philosophy and to remember that science, being essentially "open," these known limits are always the present one.

K. Jaspers, whom we have quoted in this conclusion has little belief in scientific psychology, because as a former psychiatrist he has contributed to the distinction between "explaining" and "understanding" and neglected to follow, in psychology itself, the way in which these two concepts tend to become interdependent instead of excluding each other as was formerly the case. But if he does not believe that psychology exhausts human nature, it is for two reasons against which there are no arguments: science takes no account of freedom [2] and the relationship to God. If he believes in a *philosophia perennis*, which consists "in opening our being to its innermost depths" (p. 10), and if he is of the opinion that neither human nature extended in the perspective of the two beliefs just noted, nor "the universal being in its totality," are an "object of knowledge" (p. 107), the limits which he thus assigns to science are for him in fact those of all knowledge. Often, he says, the originators of great metaphysical systems "have assumed that these systems give us objective knowledge, when seen from this point of view they are completely false" (p. 41).

We do not quote Jaspers because we accept his metaphysics, but merely give him as an example of a "wisdom," unfortunately rarely met with, and what is much more surprising, as Professor of Philosophy since 1921 (at Heidelberg, then at Bale), Jaspers taught that philosophy does not progress (p. 2) in opposition to science. Between an existentialism which in conformity with its internal logic shows itself in a rational *praxis*, and scientific research there would thus be no conflict as regards principles. The conflict would, on the contrary, remain wholly on the field of *praxis* itself, between those taking up such an approach and those who prefer somewhat more progressive ideals.

One can finally ask if the opposition between scientists and philosophers does not often depend on the fact itself that science constantly progresses, despite its crises and temporary deadends, while the way of philosophy consists in constantly readjusting to a certain number of essential and almost permanent positions to the state of knowledge at a specific time, but always after it has been sifted and generally accepted. This would explain, on the one hand, the rarity of great philosophers compared with the number of innovators in all the particular fields of science. But it would above all explain the lack of understanding that the common sense of average philosophers shows (with respect to disciplines which are in a state of continual develop-

---

[2] We have seen in Chapter Two (under A) that this statetment is perhaps no longer true.

ment, since their understanding of them, obtained solely from the reading of texts, is from this fact alone constantly being out-dated.[3] In this sense the disagreement could still continue for a long time, unless there was a radical reform of philosophical teaching that would allow students beginning their philosophical studies the opportunity of being introduced to the very practice of scientific inquiry. In this respect the future pattern of such studies is perhaps to be found in the solution adopted in Holland of a philosophical training in interfaculty institutes, where collaboration results from actual personal contact and not merely from the comparison of texts and concepts.

As for the future of scientific psychology and other sciences concerned with problems of the mind, one should not be too pessimistic about them. Not only is their development irreversible, but it is, as in all science, an irreversibility of a particular type. Thus as R. Oppenheimer liked to say, the latter is based on a consciousness of errors that will no longer be made, for in science it is not possible to be deceived twice in the same fashion. The infinite openness of these young sciences on to new problems as well as this capacity for irreversible self-correction are hence adequate guarantees of their vitality.

[3] It is striking to see, for example, how Mueller's *L'histoire de psychologie* does not show much appreciation of scientific progress.

Postscript
to the Second Edition

THIS LITTLE BOOK arose from the growing concern caused by the odd sight of contemporary philosophy, and from the pressing need to break the silence which for many reasons, psychologically explicable but morally of little validity, surrounds this question. Philosophers have for long believed that they have the right to speak of every question without making use of methods of verification, and this is not a new phenomenon.[1] But it is a much more serious matter if they take the results of their reflections as a form of knowledge, and even as a higher form. What is surprising is that scientists belonging to the younger disciplines are not more critical of such a program, which up to now has achieved little. When philosophers increasingly attack science itself, with a severity directly (and not inversely) proportional to the square of the distances that separate them from it, one has a duty to be critical of them. This is why I thought I ought to write about this matter with much more conviction, since it is of special concern to psychologists who find their investigations duplicated by a so-called philosophical psychology, the achievements of which, as a systematic examination readily shows, have up to now been nonexistent.

Starting almost alone in this fight, without even the help of a Sancho Panza with his sense of reality, I have thought it wise to write this book so that it had the form of a personal confession and I have tried to preserve as much as possible the char-

---

[1] In respect to the relations between thought and brain, Galen had already said twenty-one centuries ago, "One will excuse philosophers withdrawn in their corner for deceiving themselves in this respect, but . . . etc." Quoted by G. Galifret, *Raison présente*, I, p. 76 (Paris).

acter of a lived experience. I have so much enjoyed writing these pages that instead of preserving a calm and ironic detachment, I allowed myself to be drawn into using immoderate language by trying to answer in advance the severe criticisms I anticipated. Further, once the book appeared I had the anxious feeling that I had been somewhat imprudent and would pay the price of my boldness if not frankness.

I have, on the contrary, been extremely surprised by the kind welcome in general which this essay has received. It has from the very first been received with interest, which was not necessarily to be expected. This postscript is written twenty months after the appearance of the first edition, and after a printing that seemed to me to be too large (it has also been translated into English, Italian, and Portuguese). I have had much support from nonphilosophers, for the most part from workers in the biological and human sciences, showing that they shared my doubts about the authenticity of philosophical knowledge. But above all, those philosophers whom I esteem most have discussed this work objectively and constructively, and have often even actively encouraged me,[2] showing that they too were aware that this was a real problem today and that the epistemology of philosophical knowledge requires to be generally reconsidered. I would therefore like to make some supplementary remarks here in order to clear up certain ambiguities.

I. The main thesis of this work is that philosophy does not give us knowledge, as it lacks methods of verification (the discovery and use of these gives *ipso facto* to all progress in the cognitive field the character of a specialized science). On the other hand, by coordinating cognitive values with other human values it can give rise to a "wisdom," but a wisdom presupposes an engagement and therefore several wisdoms nonreducible to each other can co-exist, while a single truth is alone acceptable

[2] In the *Bulletin de l'Université de Toulouse* (1966, p. 401), R. Blanché concludes with this acute psychological remark: "A disenchantment," he says, referring to Chapter One of my book, "which does not prevent M. Piaget from retaining a certain fondness for philosophy; what he has more difficulty in tolerating is the agrégé in philosophy."

when we deal with a problem of knowledge in the strict sense.

Two important objections have been made against this radical position. One of them simply forbids me to make any extrapolation as to the future, the other consists in emphasizing the rational character of a coordination of values. The use of reason, then, implies some share in truth (or knowledge), while a wisdom without truth will end in a subjective fog.

The first of these objections has been made by J. C. Piguet, the ablest of contemporary philosophers in French-speaking Switzerland, whose bold metaphysical mind made me expect a more critical response.[3] "I believe that it is necessary to agree with M. Piaget on the *question of fact*. For philosophy in the past has never ended in knowledge in the true sense of the word. It has claimed to be knowledge, but it has not given us knowledge. . . . But it does not follow from this (and this is now the *question of principle*) that philosophy ought to stop aspiring to knowledge. . . . Methodologically, one cannot necessarily infer from the fact that philosophy has failed in its cognitive task that it *ought* always to fail. . . . Meanwhile, the major problem which awaits the philosophy of tomorrow is that of its own method: M. Piaget has convinced us of this." Formulated thus, this objection is irrefutable. If one has not the right to anticipate the future of science, as I have constantly stressed, as against positivism, it is only right to refrain equally from all predictions with respect to philosophy. When J. C. Piguet reminds us that algebra has taken "at least three centuries" to become established, my only comment is that we have, on the other hand, waited twenty-five centuries for a philosophical methodology. We would therefore be ill-advised not to agree tacitly to renew its lease of life for another such period.

Meanwhile I have spoken of "wisdom" or of a "rational coordination of values," and many objections have been made here, for, concerned above all to defend knowledge, I may have given the impression that there is a radical opposition between

[3] *Cahiers protestants*, 1966, 2, pp. 49–55.

wisdom and truth. In a sympathetic review [4] of my "book sometimes irritating always salutary," J. Lacroix says, for example: "the feeling remains . . . that this 'rational faith' in which philosophy consists arises uniquely from individual opinions and cannot claim any type of universality. Since these wisdoms have nothing to do with truth they could not be validly communicated." To which Lacroix adds that in a Kantian fashion he would prefer to regard philosophy as a "rational belief."

Two complementary answers can be given to J. Lacroix's objection, often repeated since. The first is that if one wished to establish the closest possible connections between wisdom and reason, which both of us desire (and "my" wisdom can be described as "rational belief" as much as "his"), one has, nevertheless, to recognize the existence of irrationalist trends in philosophy and in particular in contemporary philosophy. It is the impossibility of excluding these trends that forces us, if we wish to remain objective, to give a definition of philosophy wide enough to include them. I personally experience a complete aversion with respect to existentialism, which blurs all values and degrades man by reducing freedom to arbitrary choice and thought to self-affirmation, but I am honestly forced to recognize a philosophy in it. "Thought only begins," says Heidegger, "when we shall have learned that Reason, which has been so exaggerated over the centuries, is the most inveterate enemy of thought." [5] Let this be so for Heidegger, for certain of Jaspers' works, and for their followers. We have here, therefore, an example of a nonrational "wisdom," and I have no right to exclude it from philosophy.

Secondly, I will argue that the only difference between wisdoms having a rational character and systems of "knowledge" is that they add two supplementary elements to the latter: (1) a factor of decision or of engagement, which alone is able to give a "meaning" to life and man; and (2) a set of hypotheses which can become knowledge once they are demonstrated, but

---

[4] *Le Monde*, 31 December, 1965.
[5] Quoted by V. Leduc, *Raison présente*, I, p. 9.

if one wishes to live according to the "meaning" adopted, one is forced to accept them as beliefs without waiting for this verification. In this respect all the intermediaries are possible between the extremes of wisdom and knowledge, therefore between philosophy and science: a "wisdom" consisting of 99% knowledge and 1% of decision and belief, a "wisdom" consistting of 98% of the former and 2% of the latter, etc. These percentages are merely meant to show the impossibility of setting up *in fact* a radical opposition between wisdom and knowledge, whereas *in principle* honesty forces me to admit that if I believe without a shadow of doubt in human freedom, it is still a matter of wisdom and not of knowledge, even when verification will perhaps be possible one day.

II. In the perspective of rational wisdoms to which we are limiting ourselves, many other questions can be raised, and P. Ricoeur has done this with his usual penetration in a debate at the *Union rationaliste*,[6] where he began the discussion by starting from points of agreement in order to try to show that they imply that which I would have wished to deny. Let us therefore accept the notion of wisdom as a coordination of values, Ricoeur says: this implies at first that this question has a *meaning*, and if there is a coordination then there is *thought* and *reason*, otherwise we fall back into irrationalism; if there is reason, there is the possibility of a truth that transcends knowledge in the strict sense. Ricoeur agrees that the latter is dependent upon verification either in its experimental or deductive technical sense, but there remain the questions of preliminary conditions and of meaning, and we are then in the field of philosophical thought, which is reflective, *i.e.* arising from a third type of truth: reflection is "the grasping of the meaning of all those concepts starting from which it is possible that there be "man" (p. 58).

We are now at the very heart of the problem. I will, however, continue along the same lines as Ricoeur by asking in my

6 *Raison présente*, I, pp. 51–78.

turn new preliminary questions: what is the "meaning of meaning" and what are the truth conditions on the basis of which one can speak validly of the conditions of knowledge or truth?

I have already dealt with the question of reason. To be sure, the coordination of values or beliefs presupposes reason and thought. But reason goes beyond knowledge, since it can enter into a decision. To assert that the beliefs making up a wisdom imply reason does not mean that they give us knowledge, unless one introduces a reflective truth different from experimental knowledge or logic, and this we will come to later.

The main problem is then that of the "meaning of meaning." I believe that this fundamental concept of "meaning," which is at the center of all contemporary philosophical reflection, hides a no less important ambiguity. Ricoeur refers to Kant, the father of us all, and states the problem of man as a function of three questions: What can I know? What ought I to do? What can I hope for? But we have here two extremes of meaning: that of epistemological meaning and that of vital, or praxic, meaning. For example, has the assertion of freedom a meaning? From the epistemological point of view it certainly has one: it is the hypothesis according to which state $t + 1$ cannot be immediately inferred from state t, etc., and there is a set of physical, psychological, and logico-mathematical meanings (Gödel's theorem, etc.), which gives a clear meaning to the problem, even if it cannot perhaps yet be solved to everyone's satisfaction. From the point of view of *praxis, i.e.* from that of what man ought to do and can hope for, freedom naturally also involves a "meaning" that engages all our responsibility. But these two "meanings" cannot be reduced to each other: the inference starting from the second does not enable us to solve the epistemological problem and the inference starting from the first is not sufficient to guarantee the second. This is why, incidentally, we need a "wisdom" to coordinate them without it enabling us, as such, to attain knowledge or even "truth."

In short, a "meaning" and, moreover, "for man" has always at least two meanings, one cognitive and the other vital. It seems to me that one plays a little too easily on words in wishing to combine them into a single concept of "meaning," however close they may be in certain cases.

In the case of reflective "truth," *i.e.* one having an epistemological "meaning," let us return to the preliminary problems. This comes to asking what are the conditions of a valid analysis of conditions, therefore what are the necessary and sufficient epistemological conditions for there to be an epistemology of meaning? In this respect reflection, although obviously "necessary," remains a method that is far from being "sufficient," and hence we need to mistrust the kinds of "truths" to which they can lead.

First, the question of fact. Plato, Descartes, Leibniz, Kant and Husserl have all used "reflection." How are we then to explain the surprising differences between their epistemologies? Can a truth without universal consensus deserve to be called a truth, even if one postulates a third category in addition to experimental and deductive knowledge?

Next, the question of principle. Reflection either precedes experimentation and deduction so as to suggest the latter, or it occurs after them in order to judge and give them a "meaning." Is it then legitimate to see in this a third independent source of knowledge or is it not rather a substitute form of functioning of the whole of the cognitive operations, in the limited extent in which they constantly tend to transcend themselves in order to construct a new level of reflective abstraction? [7] This is the central question and the analysis of "reflective abstraction" in history as in psychogenesis shows that the powers of reflection, al-

---

[7] I have also called "reflective abstraction" the mode of abstraction that derives its knowledge not from objects as in the case of simple abstraction, but from actions and from the subject's operations. It is reflective in the twofold sense of the word, in a quasi-physical sense in that it reflects (like a light-ray) on to a higher level what it derives from a lower level, and in the cognitive sense of mental reflection. Thus defined, reflective abstraction is necessarily constructive and enlarges and enriches the structures from which it starts, reconstructing them on a conceptual level, and in this way ends at new structures, which are now operational in character, and are no longer due to the simple reflection from which they originated.

though considerable and always important, are inseparable from this twofold activity of experimental objectification and of internal and deductive decentration that characterizes the construction of knowledge.

In Chapter Three of my book (under E) I have tried to show that "intuition" in general was complex and characteristic of the initial and insufficiently analyzed phases of knowledge, that it involves a lack of differentiation between the given facts and the subject's norms, and then later on necessarily separates out into experimental knowledge and formalized deduction. A *forteriori*, this similarly holds of philosophical intuition, including that which Husserl believes to be connected with phenomena insofar as they are the indissociable product of subject and object. Now, the position of "reflection," although very different, involves certain analogous characteristics. It is different because as against intuition, whose role decreases with the progress of knowledge, reflection is necessary at all levels and even develops with this progress. But nevertheless, it exhibits this similarity of also involving a necessary connection with experiment and deduction, and therefore of gradually becoming more specialized in these two fields, especially in the use of deduction on a conceptual level. In short, reflection is necessary, but it is only a substitute, *i.e.* it constantly displaces its point of application without being self-sufficient, not having its own methods of verification. It thus necessarily tends to adopt those of experimental verification or technical deductive validation.

We cannot therefore regard reflective "truth" as a third kind of knowledge comparable to experiment or deduction; on the philosophical field it is just as complex as intuition, and this is shown by the development of epistemology itself. Initially philosophical in nature, as long as it remained purely reflective, it has now become increasingly concerned with the manner in which facts are tested by means of historico-critical and socio- or psychogenetic methods, and deductive validation as well as logical formalization. Epistemology is the best contemporary example of a discipline concerned with "meaning" and the preliminary conditions of knowledge which, from being at first purely philosophical, increasingly takes on the characteristics of a scientific inquiry, interdisciplinary in general, but not as such "metaphysical" in the traditional sense.

III. If my reflections on "wisdom" and the impossibility of maintaining two sorts of truth, one philosophical and the other scientific, has, as was expected, thus given rise to all sorts of objections, I have, however, been much struck by the silence, sometimes approving but sometimes embarrassed, with which my criticisms of "philosophical psychology" have been received. The reasons for this are clear. While the philosophers of the Faculty of Letters of Geneva try to revive this declining discipline (I have taken this example from where I have been able to find it, since such tendencies opposed to the general trend of intellectual progress are becoming increasingly rare), the teaching of psychology in the Faculty of Letters and even in the philosophy sections is increasingly becoming directed toward experimental research, in France at the present time as much as elsewhere.[8] The psychologists of the Sorbonne have even recently established a separate subsection from that of the philosophers, etc.

In the *Union rationaliste* debate to which I have already referred, J. P. Sartre was defended by his friend F. Jeanson. I very much enjoyed his witty and biting remarks in criticizing

[8] In a semi-official publication, the report prepared for UNESCO, *Les Sciences de l'homme en France* (prepared by Jean Viet, Mouton 1966; no. 7 of the *Publications du Conseil International des Sciences Sociales*), we read (pp. 78–79): "However, if it appears that philosophy increasingly takes account of the contributions of psychology, of sociology . . . (etc.), it is a fact that studies in the different sciences of man tend at the present time in France to become separated from philosophy. It is clear, for example, that psychologists today are more sympathetic to modeling their discipline on the exact and natural sciences than to fitting it into the philosophical perspective opened up by Husserl's phenomenology. . . . One notes, moreover, the position adopted in ethnology by C. Levi-Strauss which ends if not in rejecting, at least in a kind of bracketing of philosophy. The widening gap between the sciences of man and philosophy appears greater still if one abstracts from the former certain disciplines which traditionally form part of it, like epistemology and logic . . . etc."

me for having taken as a target Sartre's studies on emotion and imagery, as if this were a too easy task and as if it were self-evident that these studies were somewhat outdated and hardly accepted by Sartre today. At which Fraisse asked him to bring this fact to the notice of a wider audience, bearing in mind the dissertation subjects which the agrégés in philosophy give to their students, as in these quarters "Sartre's theory of emotions is still fashionable. If Sartre and the Sartrians tell us that this youthful essay is now outdated much time would be saved in the philosophy classes in this institution (the meeting took place at the Sorbonne)" (p. 66).

Fraisse continued by showing that if Ravaisson and Bergson have spoken of habit, all our present knowledge of the subject is due to laboratory experiments. If Bergson gave a brilliant critique of psycho-physics, he told us nothing about the relationships between the sensations that we experience and the external physical stimuli, while psycho-physics has successfully continued its work and has given rise to numerous applications. Merleau-Ponty has dealt with size-constancy in speaking "ably about our work, but without introducing anything new," etc.

G. Galifret has recalled Bergson's theory of memory "of which fortunately neuro-physiology has never taken any notice" (p. 76) and he shared Fraisse's surprise that the philosophers present "should have quickly dropped philosophical psychology which ought, however, to be at the very center of our discussions; I would add that if no one wants to defend it, perhaps it is because this kind of psychology is indefensible" (p. 68).

While the public debate from which I have taken these extracts ought to have been concerned with "psychology and philosophy" and with replying to my criticisms of philosophical psychology, Ricoeur alone among the philosophers remarked that scientific psychology would not be able to work without a philosophical problem, which brings us back to the question of "meaning." To this I would reply by distinguishing the subject-psychologist who constructs his science, and any human subject whatsoever, the object of the psychologist's studies. The subject-psychologist constructs his epistemology as a function of the progress or the turning points of his science, and especially as a function of the increasing number of relationships between it and other disciplines. There is therefore no need for the philosopher to intervene at a higher level in order to construct a complete epistemology, since the latter develops itself as a function of the growing complexity of the psychologist's own investigations and the conceptual advance they entail. As long as it is a question of epistemological "meaning," the sciences are self-sufficient and alone guarantee their own "reflection."

As for the human subject in general, this is an entirely different matter, for he uses norms of every kind, cognitive, ethical, etc. He is engaged in the world and attributes to everything a "meaning" from vital, social, or personal, as well as epistemological points of view. If the concept of "meaning" can be given a global significance, it particularly applies in the case of the "average" human subject. What needs to be strongly emphasized is that it is the subject himself in his interpersonal relationships and in his own spontaneity who is the origin of these "meanings" and not the philosopher or the psychologist. The question then is, who is in a better position to give us a theory of meaning in its human context: the philosopher who sees things from on high, or the psychologist and psycho-sociologist whose precise function is to try to understand how the subject (the human subject and not the psychologist) elaborates these norms? I believe that in the field of cognitive norms we have learned more by studying how the "meaning" of rational operations develops from birth to adult age, than by reference to philosophical epistemologies. Why should things be different with respect to the different kinds of "meaning" not exclusively epistemological?

In a discussion at the *Centre d'Etudes européennes*, Jeanne Hersch stated: "for those who want to remain on the purely empirical level, who wish, for example, to reduce man to an object of objective studies of a psychological or biological or sociological kind, the expression 'all men are equal' has not in my opinion any meaning." [9] This advice is to be welcomed if it recommends us not to prescribe norms relating to equality in terms of bio-psycho-sociological considerations, but it is quite useless, since we are not as naive as all this. If, on the other hand, it means that men experience themselves as active, free, and responsible, and attach a value or a particular "meaning" to the idea of equality, that the philosopher is better qualified than we are to understand how the subject has arrived at this idea, then we need to note that it is not the philosopher who creates "meaning" but man insofar as he is a subject. Then why bring in the philosopher? The honest psychologist or sociologist who, without at all wishing to prescribe for or against equality, studies how this concept results from a noninnate tendency but one that increasingly manifests itself during the development of the child or of certain societies, may perhaps throw fresh light on this norm instead of stating on a higher level what everyone knows in advance (since we are all subjects and we even at times try to "reflect").

IV. I now come to the most contentious part of my study, i.e. to Chapter Five, where I have tried to show by precise examples how philosophers behave when they approach factual problems using the method of simple reflection and without that training which makes experimentalists wish to employ verification, even in the case of hypotheses that appear to be forced upon us by immediate deduction starting from already verified facts. In discussing these examples, it seemed to me that I ought to enter into some detail, for it is useless simply to state in general terms the dangers of purely reflective incursions in questions arising from experience. It is only by examining closely the structure of an argument that one observes its soundness. I have specifically quoted from certain discussions in which I have been involved, since I was then able to deal with facts with which I was well acquainted. I have in this case been accused of singling out for attack my fellow-countrymen, and engaging in controversy with close colleagues. I do not at all see why I

[9] *L'Europe et le monde*, Vol. XI, 1966, p. 44.

should not reply to questions in which I have been personally involved, especially if this discussion can help to show how philosophers approach questions of science or verification. But in examining some of the reactions that my replies have produced (with, I recognize, some stylistic exuberance bordering on rudeness), I have observed this fact, still very general, which it may be instructive to note. The ordinary person finds it quite natural that philosophers should criticize an experimental result, as if the higher level of their reflections gives them the right to have a universal outlook; while if the scientist or the psychologist whose conclusions have been treated as "singularly dangerous" or accused of an "empty universality," replies by querying the very method of investigation or of discussion of the philosopher, one tends to see in this a reversal of positions and values, which is suspect if not a kind of intellectual high treason.

It may be useful to begin by mentioning, even when it is not yet a question of "facts" but still of the attitude of the philosopher toward science in general, an interesting objection that has been made to me in connection with the philosophy of F. Brunner, whose theocentrism and somewhat superficial remarks on the "naive naturalism of science" has made me speak of "Brunnerocentrism" in a little note which was to be taken more as a caricature than seriously. Brunner, who is a charming person, has reacted with spirit, and one of his defenders has raised the following general problem: "The fact that metaphysics understood in this sense is not everyone's concern does not authorize us to conclude that it is not knowledge. Higher mathematics is also restricted to a small group of individuals. Why not admit that in order to be a metaphysician one needs to have aptitudes in the same way as it is necessary to have them in order to be a mathematician?" It is assumed that the answer given to this question can explain why the metaphysician feels he has the right to speak from on high of the sciences with which, however, he is ill-acquainted. But the difficulty remains to explain why, if I have not the necessary aptitudes to understand mathematical and physical theories, I still do not question them, while the metaphysics of St. Anselm or of F. Brunner can leave me puzzled. In addition to the problem of aptitude there therefore enters a question of belief, and the characteristic of a belief is precisely that it is not regarded as knowledge by those who do not share it. Have we then to admit that it is this belief itself that characterizes the presupposed aptitude? But Kant's example shows that one can proceed from dogmatism to criticism in conserving one's beliefs while modifying one's epistemological positions. And in connecting aptitude and belief, one then ends with a hierarchy of systems, of which certain privileged ones form the apex while others permanently remain at the base. Writers on the latter level thus may with reason form the impression in this case, of what I termed with some maliciousness Brunnerocentrism.

R. Ruyer has sent me a long letter the objectivity and generosity of which filled me with embarrassment and admiration. If I understand him rightly we share the twofold conviction of the impossibility of a specifically philosophical knowledge and of the need to look for the origins of the "subject" on the biological plane. It is this lively awareness of the interdependency of the biological and the mental which makes him speak of "absolute" domains, in the sense that they do not need an observer or an external agent to be observed. But why then in spite of the sympathy which the experimentalist cannot but have for the idea of a psycho-biological synthesis, which pervades Ruyer's work, why is it that the experimentalist cannot help but have certain misgivings on then seeing him pass so rapidly through the stages leading from the amoeba to the human brain? On reading Ruyer's letter I would have been tempted—and I say this in all sincerity—to state in this postscript that I had completely misunderstood him and that he is in the right. And I ask myself again what are the chief reasons preventing me from doing this. Perhaps (and I do not exclude this from being the most frequent cause of the tragic divorce between philosophers and experimentalists) it is simply that R. Ruyer already knows what the "subject" is, while we continue to seek it.[10] Is the essential characteristic of the subject at all levels to know or observe himself, or is this a very derivative form of conduct, by relation to *what he does*, without his yet being able to know that he does it? We are faced with such doubts almost on every page of his work.

My discussion with R. Schaerer has, if I may say so, ended excellently (and this is due to him alone). After taking up again the discussion in the *Journal de Genève*, for which he writes on philosophy, Schaerer has closed it by a brief article that gave satisfaction to all. On the one hand, he denied to the philosopher "by a categorical *no* . . . the right to have a say in matters of fact which arise from specialized science"; but on the other hand he takes up again the point that all scientific activity occurs "in a wider universe which is that of moral conduct, of the meaning of life, or final ends, and which in short necessarily brings up the problem of 'meaning.' " We have dealt with this question above (under II) and need not return to it, especially as Schaerer explicitly refers here to the vital meaning and not to the epistemological.

I have considered still other examples in Chapter Five, one of which was Bergson's unfortunate encounter with the theory of relativity. Not everyone has approved of them, and a historian of philosophy has stated that Bergson has shown great intellectual honesty in finally withdrawing his book (on this topic) from his collected works. This is not the time to reopen the

[10] "The scientific investigator who begins an experiment," Galifret rightly remarks, *Raison présente*, I, p. 69, "does not know where the experiment will lead him; he hopes to verify his hypothesis but at the same time he hopes for the unexpected, the unusual, germ of a new hypothesis richer in explanatory value. The vicissitudes of this enterprise are the elements of a dialogue in which, if it is the investigator who questions, it is the experiment which has the last word. It seems to me that the philosopher's procedures are entirely different and are almost opposite in character. The philosopher often gives the impression of starting from the conclusion and endeavoring with more or less verbal fluency to persuade people of it. He does not approach the truth by successive approximations. A choice having been made he has to defend it. . . ."

discussion and introduce distinctions between an honesty forced upon one and spontaneous doubts. I merely want to say that in connection with this question of philosophers involving themselves in problems of fact, I have received much more support than I had expected from a number of philosophers acutely aware of the dangers of the present situation, and this from very different quarters (from the Sorbonne to the Pontifical University of Rome). One may therefore hope that the links between philosophy and science will be renewed when the phenomenological and existentialist fashion in philosophy will have waned.

The great remedy for the illusion of the directive or at least synthetic role which some philosophers still want to play, is the growing development of interdisciplinary relationships between the specialized sciences. For long the rule in the natural sciences, such relationships are becoming increasingly common in the human sciences, and it is clear that interdisciplinary progress in a question which a particular science cannot itself solve will weaken merely "reflective" considerations and favor experimental investigations or the appearance of new positive facts. It might be worthwhile to note by way of an example that after a congress of French-speaking philosophers on the topic of language (Geneva, 1966), a discussion took place on the two levels of meaning distinguished by Benveniste. The linguist R. Gödel then concluded as follows: [11] "Linguists are today interested above all in system, that is to say in the first stage of meaning. As to the passage of the first to the second,[12] enlightenment will come, I think, from experimental psychology. As for philosophers, I doubt whether they have anything important to say on this question." In quoting the above, I do not, however, want to assert that this is the necessary balance sheet of a philosophical congress.

V. We must conclude this retrospective survey of a work which is perhaps self-sufficient, but whose defects as well as good points I have seen more clearly after having had the comments

---

[11] *Journal de Genève*, 13 September 1966, p. 13.
[12] *Cf*. The problems of speech as opposed to those of language.

of the many readers who were kind enough to communicate them to me.

I ought to have developed this conclusion in the body of the work itself, since I recounted my experiences there and since everyone can see from my account what I have in fact obtained from my philosophical training. I have derived from it nothing less than the general set of problems that has directed my later studies, and this is a considerable debt; only—and it is this second aspect that I have particularly stressed, for it is less obvious —I have only been able to approach the solution of the problems thus stated by abandoning the reflective methods of the philosopher in order to base my work on experiment and more or less formalized deduction.

In broad outline, a lived experience has nothing singular about it; it only reflects the actual tendencies occurring in one's formative environment. We need therefore have no fear in generalizing the scope of the two preceding findings. In fact the whole history of modern philosophy is that of problems raised by reflection but not solved by it, and those which have received a solution have first had to be transferred from the philosophical field to that of the specialized sciences which have developed from it by progressive differentiation. I have tried to give several examples of this in Chapter Two. In the article quoted above J. C. Piguet has himself given an excellent example, that of "continuity," anticipated by Nicholas of Cusa but demonstrated only by Leibniz in his mathematical work.[13]

[13] "M. Piaget is of the general opinion that in the best of cases philosophy can *serve* the interests of science . . . in two ways: one anticipatory and the other reflective. According to the first, philosophy anticipates intuitively certain scientific results: thus Nicholas of Cusa . . . affirms continuity in nature, but it was left to Leibniz (and to Leibniz the mathematician) to *demonstrate* continuity, by inventing the infinitesimal calculus. It is one thing merely to affirm continuity in some way as "seen by the mind" (even if it was that of a genius), and it is quite another to demonstrate it in inventing at the same time not only the infinitesimal calculus, but the whole of modern dynamics, by mechanical methods. In the first case there is only an anticipation of knowledge (which others will realize as a science), in the second case there is effective knowledge, established and verifiable."

In short, philosophy, due to its reflective method, raises problems, but does not solve them, because reflection does not by itself involve methods of verification. The sciences by their use of the methods of experimentation and deduction solve some problems and constantly give rise to new ones, but without the initial impulse due to reflection on problems as a whole; and doubtless without the renewed stimulus of continuous reflection, scientific problems would probably be more limited. This does not mean, however, that they would conform to the narrow ideal that positivism and empiricism have wanted to give to them. It is of little importance whether we restrict the term "philosophy" only to that of philosophers, or also include that of scientists who "reflect," and whether we restrict the term "science" to scientists alone or include the great philosophers who have known how to experiment and to make deductions (cf. Chapter Two); all this is unimportant. What is important is the trilogy reflection $\times$ deduction $\times$ experiment, the first term representing the heuristic function and the other two cognitive verification, which is alone constitutive of "truth."

But there remain problems that science cannot solve either temporarily or in some cases can only solve on a provisional basis, which no doubt will remain final. These problems can be of vital importance and have a "meaning" according to the second of the two meanings distinguished above. They therefore require equally "provisional" solutions, the word "provisional" dating from Descartes. To want to consider them as modes of knowledge is a constantly recurring illusion of some philosophers. But in interpreting them as a wisdom (or, since the solutions are numerous and irreducible, as "wisdoms"), and as wisdoms as rational and as basic to "knowledge" as one would wish, the agreement between knowledge and praxis will no longer be disturbed by the interventions of philosophers, which can only damage the one as much as the other.

Index

'accident', 124, 126, 128
affectivity, 159, 199
Anglo-Saxon ideological tradition, 54
anthropology, philosophical, 15, 23, 38, 71, 204–5
a priori structuring, 50ff, 56–8, 73, 81
argumentation, 63, 65
Aristotelian biology, 45, 47f; epistemology, 50; physics, 181–2; theory of forms, 48f
assimilation, 8, 97, 131–2, 149f, 159
association, 150, 159, 196, 199f
atomism, 149
autonomy, 190ff

Bachelard, G., 24, 166, 169
Bachelard, S., 82, 169
behavior and consciousness, 156f, 159f, 198
Bergson, H., 5f, 9, 83f, 145, 224; fundamental antitheses, 89–101; intuition, 86, 88, 112, 139, 141; philosophical psychology, 124, 150–2, 154, 163; relativity, 92, 171, 175–7, 229
Beth, E. W., 25, 33f, 105
Binet, A., 9, 28, 135, 137, 196, 199f
biology, 45, 47ff, 177f; and nature of life, 206f; and philosophy 78, 179, 184ff, 228–9; Élements de psychobiologie, 184; molecular, 83, 93

Biran, Maine de, and causality, 145–50; introspection, 143–5; metaphysical psychology, 84–86; philosophical psychology, 123f, 150
biunivocal correspondence, 126f
Brentano, F. C., 130, 172
British philosophers, viii–ix
Brunner, F., 117n, 227
Brunschvicg, L., 9f, 17, 61, 74, 101f, 121, 148, 169–70
Buytendijk, F. J. J., 134n, 142

causality, 40, 50, 85, 136, 143, 145–9
Cassirer, E., 61
Cavailles, J., 105, 169
centration and decentration, 111, 115, 142–3, 149, 222
Centre international d'épistémologie génétique, 30–1, 33, 35–7, 127; symposia, 33–4, 37
chance, 93, 179
Claparède, E., 8, 10, 125, 134f, 137f, 200
Comte, A., 17, 40
consciousness, 40, 133–8, 154–6, 158f, 160f, 188, 195, 198; stream of, 101, 150, 155
continuity in nature, 231f
coordination of values, 3–4, 59–61, 84, 207, 211, 217ff
Cuénot, L., 180, 182, 185
cybernetics, 41f, 93, 99, 136, 184

Dalbiez, R., 180–4, 188, 190
de Beauregard, Costa, 37, 90
deduction, 20, 83, 111, 167, 222, 232
deductive analysis, 73
Descartes, R., 46f, 50–4 *pass*., 72; and causality, 145; and reflection, 221
dialectical knowledge, 111, 115–16, 204; materialism, 39–40
directed passage, 190–1, 192f
duration, lived, 94f, 171, 175

effort, 143–6
egocentrism, 190, 192
eidetic knowledge, 109–12 *pass*.
Einstein, A., 83, 112f, 167, 176f
empiricism, 31f, 51–6, 74f, 127
epistemological and individual subject, 55ff, 170
epistemology, 7–8, 10, 35, 48, 71–6, 83, 201, 222, 225; and Aristotle, 47ff; and Descartes, 50f, 54; compartmentalization, 61–2; delimitation of problems, 72–7; genetic, vii, 24, 28–9, 34f, 75
equilibrium, 185; and reversibility, 193f, 201–2
essences, 124–6, 128, 142
ethics, 66–8
evolution, 49, 95, 180
existentialism, 86f, 218
experience, 54ff, 75, 85, 202f, 226; originary, 155–64 *pass*.
experimental interpretation, 111, 226
experimentation, 127, 167f, 221f, 232

facts: and philosophy, 165–7, 169, 176, 226–30 *pass*.; and psychology, 124–8, 141f, 167; and science, 120–1
finality, 40, 42, 50, 78–80, 179–83, 185; models simulating, 93, 100, 193

Flournoy, T., 13, 22, 164
Fraisse, P., 27, 163, 188, 224
France, psychology studies in, 24–8
Frege, G., 23, 59, 72, 104, 126
Freud, S., 152, 198
Freudianism, 159
functionalism, American, 196

Galifret, G., 224, 229n
games, theory of, 67
Gestalt theory, 23, 102, 159, 196, 200–1
Gödel, K., 41, 74
Gödel, R., 230
Godot, Paul, 4
Godot, Pierre, 13
Goldmann, L., 13, 65, 169, 204
Gonseth, F., 19, 33f, 92, 127; *idonéisme*, 166
Granger, C. G., 37, 169, 205n
Gréco, P., 35
Grize, J. B., 35, 37, 189
groups, theory of, 113
Gurwitsch, Aron, 109, 131
Guye, C. E., 82f, 90, 179

Hegel, G. W. F., 47, 58, 86, 115
Heidegger, Martin, 218; Being and language, 118–20
Helmholtz, H. L. F. von, 73, 90
Hersch, Jeanne, 37f, 225
heteronomy, 190
historico-critical method, 10f, 74f
Holland, philosophical studies in, 25, 213
Hume, David, 47, 52–5, 145–8 *pass*.
Husserl, E. G., 22, 47, 62, 91, 126, 221; anti-psychologism, 59, 70; criticism of psychology, 105–6, 109f; intentionality, 130; intersubjectivity, 138; 160; intuition, 102ff, 112f; lived world theory, 156; phenomenology, 101–11, 156; reflection, 221

idonéisme, 166
Inhelder, B., 15n, 22, 152n, 168n
innateness, 52f, 56
instinct, 95–7
intelligence, 96–100
intentionality, vii, 130–3, 141, 161f
interdisciplinary studies, 29–30, 35, 62, 230
International Council of Philosophy and Human Sciences, 206
International Institute of Philosophy, xiii, 64
International Union of Scientific Psychology, 23, 64, 123, 206
intersubjectivity, 138, 160
introspection, x, 85, 100, 124, 133, 137, 138–45 *pass.*, 195f, 199f
intuition, 19–20, 86–90 *pass.*, 96, 100–5 *pass.*, 110–15, 116, 139, 158, 165, 222
irrationalism, 86f, 140–1, 218f

James, W., 6, 22, 144, 150, 196; and stream of consciousness, 101
Janet, P., 10f, 134, 141, 144, 151f, 168, 198f
Jaspers, K., 130, 209ff, 212, 218

Kant, E., 17, 47, 56–7, 71f, 81, 85, 117, 139, 145, 220f
knowledge, distinction of philosophical and scientific, xivf, 26f, 43f, 59–62, 65, 79, 81, 87–90, 111–17, 157, 177, 210, 216ff, 228
Köhler, W., 183, 200f

Lalande, A., 9f, 20, 84
Leibniz, G. W., 39, 47, 49, 51f, 53f, 69, 72, 221, 231
Le Roy, E., 101, 176
lived world hypothesis, 156–60
Locke, John, 47, 51ff, 155
logic, 49, 55, 69f, 105

logico-mathematical deduction, 12, 32, 56, 106f, 167, intelligence, 51f, 55, 75, 99

McCulloch, W., 37, 99
Maritain, J., 171, 173–4
Marx, K., 39, 47; dialectic, 58, 203ff
materialism, 39f, 83f
Mays, W., 29, 31, 32n, 34n
meaning, concept of, 118, 130, 132, 136f, 156ff, 161, 218–21, 222, 225–6, 229, 232
memory, 151–4, 188, 224
Merleau-Ponty, M., 23f, 78, 87, 143, 224; philosophical psychology, 155–60; subjectivity, 157, 159–63
metaphysical knowledge, 41f, 63–6, 85f, 100–1
metaphysics, 83, 118ff
Metz, A., 95, 170, 176f
Meyer, F., 37, 134, 169, 178
Meyerson, E., 17, 73
Mueller, F. L., 38, 122, 195–208; on contemporary psychology, 205–8; on philosophical psychology, 133ff, 195; on Piaget, 201–4; on trends in psychology, 197–201

Næss, A., 33f
norms, 165, 191–4, 225–6

objectivist school, 96, 134n, 182
onto-genesis, 158, 185
ontology, 103, 118, 166
open systems, 90
Oxford school of linguistic philosophy, viii

Papert, S., 36, 99
parascientific philosophies, 62, 82–8
Perelman, C., 63, 65
phenomenological reduction, 105–108

phenomenology, 23, 37, 80f, 101ff, 109–11, 155, 205
philosophers' intervention in scientific fields, 17, 91, 169f, 181–3, 188, 211–13, 229, 232
philosophers, training of, viii–ix, 168–9
philosophical psychology, viii, 22, 38, 122f, 132, 162–4, 215; and Biran, 123f, 143ff, 150; and Merleau-Ponty, 155–63; and nature of man, 206–9, 225; methodology, 141f, 194f, 199, 206, 217; subject matter, 124, 133
philosophy: and criticism of science, 117–18, 227; and differentiation of science, 44–6, 60, 62, 210, 231; and methods of verification, 216; illusions of, xii, 116f, 232; moral, 66–8; trends in, 59–62
physics, transformation of, 92f
physiological psychology, 196
Piaget, J., xff, 5–10; and Mueller's views, 201–3; and philosophical psychology, 223f; and philosophy, 10–24; abstract models, 136; conceptual prolems, 126, 128; decentration, 143; genetic epistemology, 28–35, 38; intentionality, 131–3; norms of truth, 19–21; verification, 126–8
Pieron, H., 24, 28, 134
Piguet, J. C., 217, 231
Plato, 45, 47, 112, 221
Plotinus, 46f
Poincaré, H., 32, 73, 75
positivism, 17–18, 40, 42, 115, 117
pre-established harmony, 51f, 57
psychologists, training of, 24–6
psychology, experimental, 8, 10, 14, 22, 27, 72, 110; and linguists, 230
psychology, genetic, 28–35, 38, 103, 143, 196f
psychology, metaphysical, 84, 86
psychology, phenomenological, 128f, 136, 142
psychology, scientific, 18, 71, 122ff, 211, 224f; history of, 196–7; Mueller on, 195ff; neglect of consciousness, 135, 137
psychology of conduct, 134, 195f, 200
psycho-physiological parallelism, 145, 154–5

Quine, W. V., 31, 33, 37

reciprocity, 190ff
reflection, 11f, 16, 168f, 176, 189, 195, 226, 231f
reflective truth, 219–22
relativity, 8–9, 92, 95, 169–71, 173–6
Reverdin, H., 22
reversibility, 108ff, 193f, 201–2
revisability, 191
Reymond, A., 6–10 pass., 74, 170
Ricoeur, P., 219f, 224
Rockefeller Foundation, 29–30, 35
Russell, B., 30, 52, 72f, 126
Ruyer, R., 134, 183–8, 228

Sartre, J. P., 23, 89, 91, 223f; dialectic thought, 115; essences, 124–5, 128; introspection, 100, 139f; magical action, 132f, 140, 155, 161, 163
Schaerer, R., 37f, 190–4, 229
scientists and philosophy, 61, 120–1
self-regulation, 8, 99, 144, 146, 182f, 185, 193
Société romande de Philosophie, 37, 189
Society for Philosophy of Nature, 183
Spinoza, B. de, 47, 61
structures, hereditary, 55; oper-

ational, 51, 85, 106–9 *pass.*,
184–5
subjectivity, 156–7, 159–62
subject-object interaction, 102–3,
113–14
Szeminska, A., 22

technicality, 166, 169
theocentrism, 227
Thomism, 124, 130, 171, 175
transcendence, 47, 84, 104, 156,
161
transformism, 180f, 183
truth, 79–80, 210, 216–23 *pass.*,
232

Union rationaliste, 219, 223

verification, xiv, 11, 20, 125–8
pass., 138, 142, 147f, 166, 191,
194, 197, 203, 215f, 222, 228–9
vitalism, 83, 91ff, 188

Wallon, H., 28, 203
Whitehead, A. N., 30, 72f
wisdom, xiiif, 12, 44, 65, 116,
209–12 *pass.*, 216–20, 223, 232;
Kantian, 72; James's, 150
Würzburg school, 137, 196, 199

Zazzo, R., 203

Printed and bound by CPI Group (UK) Ltd, Croydon, CR0 4YY

01/11/2024

01782630-0004